THE ESSENTIAL
KIDNEY DISEASE
COOKBOOK

with **130** DELICIOUS, KIDNEY-FRIENDLY
MEALS TO MANAGE YOUR
KIDNEY DISEASE (CKD)

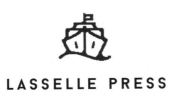

LASSELLE PRESS

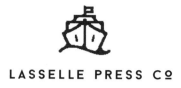

LASSELLE PRESS Co

ISBN-13:978-1911364030
ISBN-10: 1911364030

CONTENTS

CHAPTER 9
SEAFOOD | 91

CHAPTER 10
VEGETARIAN | 110

CHAPTER 11
SIDES. SALADS & SOUPS | 136

CHAPTER 12
STOCKS & SAUCES | 154

CHAPTER 13
DRINKS & DESSERTS | 166

INTRODUCTION

Welcome!

Making the decision to change your diet and lifestyle after a diagnosis of kidney disease is a huge step. You may have bought this for yourself or to help a loved one through the disease - either way, you have made the right choice.

By making the right choices along with your doctor and dietitian, it is possible to make a difference to how you feel, along with the symptoms you experience. Diet directly links to kidney disease. With the function of the kidneys being to filter out the excess waste, toxins, and liquids in your body, it's no wonder that choosing the best foods and ingredients can alleviate some of the pressure on your kidneys.

As you have bought this book, you already know that a holistic approach to treatment is so crucial and medical advice and treatment from professionals is a necessity. If you're wondering where to go next in the kitchen, this book aims to help you out.

Inside, we outline kidney disease and the different stages, along with the foods that are recommended, and those that should be cut down and even avoided in each stage.

Each recipe lists the dietary information that you should be looking out for, including phosphorous, protein and sodium. All the meals have been created to be flavorsome and healthy so that they can be enjoyed by someone with kidney disease as well as the whole family!

Thank you for purchasing this book and we hope that the information and recipes provided can help you get started, or continue, along the journey to improve your health and live well.

The Lasselle Press Team

I
KIDNEY DISEASE 101

If you have bought this book, either you or a loved one may be experiencing the symptoms caused by kidney disease. This chapter will outline the functions of the kidneys as well as some of the causes and symptoms of the disease. The good news is that if you are yet to suffer from the disease, or you're in the early stages, you can take steps to change your dietary and lifestyle habits in order to maintain healthy functioning of the kidneys for as long as possible. If you're at a later stage of kidney disease, you will have found that changing your dietary habits has become essential. This chapter aims to provide you with the information you will need to understand each stage of the disease.

YOUR KIDNEYS:

Despite their tiny size, the kidneys perform a number of functions which are vital for the body to be able to function healthily. These include:

- Filtering excess fluids and waste from the blood,
- Creating the enzyme known as renin which regulates blood pressure,
- Ensuring bone marrow creates red blood cells,
- Controlling calcium and phosphorus levels through absorption and excretion.

Unfortunately, when kidney disease reaches a chronic stage, these functions start to stop working. However, with the right treatment and lifestyle, it is possible to manage symptoms and continue living well. This is even more applicable in the earlier stages of the disease.

CAUSES OF KIDNEY DISEASE:

Unfortunately, 10% of all adults over the age of 20 will experience some form of kidney disease in their lifetime. There are a variety of different treatments for kidney disease, which depend on the cause of the disease. Possible causes are outlined below:

DIABETES: In the United States and other countries where the 'Standard American Diet' (discussed in chapter 2) runs rampant, the number one leading cause of kidney disease is high blood pressure and Type 2 diabetes. Both of these diseases are either completely preventable or at least treatable and once the root issue has been treated, kidney disease issues can also dissipate.

GLOMERULONEPHRITIS: Damage to the glomeruli (the filters in your kidneys), impairs the kidneys' ability to filter waste materials. This can be caused by damage to the immune system and if this is the case, can be treated with medication. It is either experienced for a short period of time (acute glomerulonephritis), or for a longer period of time (chronic). In chronic cases, further problems can arise such as high blood pressure, organ damage and later chronic kidney disease.

ACUTE RENAL FAILURE/ACUTE KIDNEY INJURY: Sudden damage or failure of the kidney can be caused by a rapid loss of blood to the kidneys, sepsis or even severe dehydration. Infection, poison and some medicines are also known to lead to acute kidney issues.

SUDDEN BLOCKAGE: Kidney stones, tumors, injuries and an enlarged prostate in men can stop urine from passing through the kidneys as it should. This can cause swelling in the lower extremities, a loss of appetite, vomiting or nausea, extreme tiredness, restlessness, feelings of confusion, or even an acute pain beneath the ribs (known as flank pain).

ECLAMPSIA: This can be experienced during pregnancy when the placenta doesn't function as it should do, creating high blood pressure and sometimes leading to kidney problems.

BREAKDOWN OF MUSCLE TISSUE: Under extreme pressure, for example when running a marathon or undergoing other feats of massive exertion, the body starts to break down muscle tissue after it has used all other available fuel. If this continues unchecked, too much of the protein known as myoglobin will ultimately end up in the bloodstream, putting undue strain on the kidneys and potentially leading to further implications.

IMMUNE SYSTEM: Common immune system diseases that can lead to kidney issues include lupus, hepatitis C, hepatitis B, HIV, and aids. These can lead to what is known as chronic kidney disease (any form of kidney disease that lasts for three months or longer). Sometimes the sufferer of the immune disease will not experience the symptoms of the kidney disease until it reaches a chronic stage; this can be dangerous as it is a lot harder to manage once it has reached this level.

EXTREME URINARY TRACT INFECTIONS: Urinary tract infections that occur within the kidneys rather than the bladder are known as pyelonephritis and occur when a traditional urinary tract infection remains untreated long enough for it to spread into the upper urinary tract system. This can cause scarring in the kidneys which can lead to serious flaws in kidney functioning.

STREPTOCOCCAL INFECTIONS: Commonly known as a strep infection, this bacterium can infect the throat as well as various layers of the skin, the middle ear, the sinuses or even in a more severe case, a widespread vicious rash known as scarlet fever. This bacterium is known to result in the glomeruli (individual filters in the kidneys) becoming infected.

POLYCYSTIC KIDNEY DISEASE: This type of kidney disease is typically passed down from parent to child and causes cysts filled with fluid to form on the kidneys themselves.

BIRTH DEFECTS: Depending on the severity of the defect, kidney disease could form simply because the kidneys do not function properly or because of an obstruction in the urinary tract before birth.

SYMPTOMS:

The symptoms of kidney disease vary widely and it is essential that you seek a professional diagnosis. Common symptoms below may be an indicator of the disease:

CHANGE IN URINATION PATTERNS: The most common indicator of chronic kidney disease; if you suddenly find yourself having to get up frequently at night to urinate or if the volume of urine passed significantly increases or turns pale, then you are advised to see a doctor. Likewise, if your urine becomes bubbly or foamy, contains blood, or significantly decreases in volume and turns very dark these may also be signs that the kidneys are not working as they should.

SWELLING: Chronic kidney disease means that your kidneys can not filter waste materials or liquids properly and this can result in a marked swelling of the hands, face, feet, ankles or legs. This can be particularly uncomfortable for sufferers.

FATIGUE: Healthy functioning kidneys produce erythropoietin (the hormone that moderates the oxygen levels in the blood). The disease affects the kidneys' ability to produce this hormone, thus causing a lack of oxygen in the blood. With not enough oxygen reaching the brain or other muscles in the body, lethargy and fatigue are experienced. This is a form of anemia and can be extremely debilitating if not treated properly.

RASHES: A result of streptococcal infection as outlined in the causes section.

UREMIA: Bad breath which can smell of ammonia is sometimes experienced because of the waste materials not being filtered through the kidneys effectively. If suffering from uremia, people will often find that foods they are used to eating change in taste.

VOMITING OR NAUSEA: If left untreated, uremia can also lead to nausea and vomiting over a prolonged period of time . This type of vomiting is not usually treatable with common sickness medications.

BREATHING DIFFICULTIES: Excess fluid that cannot be filtered through the kidneys can travel to the lungs, making it difficult to breathe. This can be especially problematic if experienced alongside uremia.

COLD SPELLS: Anemia can reduce blood flow to certain regions of the body and cause poor circulation. Circulation can become problematic as we age, gain weight or experience high blood pressure, however bad circulation is also a symptom of kidney disease and if you have experienced cold spells or flashes, this may be a sign of the disease.

DIZZY SPELLS: Prolonged anemia may also lead to frequent dizzy spells, making it difficult to concentrate on complicated tasks as well as impairing memory function.

LEG PAIN: Pain related to chronic kidney disease is actually felt in the kidneys themselves only a small percentage of the time. Leg pain is quite common as a result of swelling. Related issues such as bladder stones or infections as well as polycystic kidney disease are also known to cause pain in the sufferer.

5 STAGES OF KIDNEY DISEASE:

There are 5 stages of kidney disease which are measured by the glomerular filtration rate (GFR). This is calculated by a professional, according to the patient's serum creatine levels as well as their race, gender, and age. The 5 stages and their characteristics are outlined below:

STAGE 1: People with stage 1 kidney disease will have some kidney damage though their GFR will remain in the normal range. During this stage, doctors will work to determine the root of the problem so that it can best be addressed effectively. Those suffering from the disease are advised to keep their blood pressure lower than 130/80. Those who have diabetes are also encouraged to control their blood sugar levels. Regular check-ups at the doctors are essential in monitoring the disease and its symptoms.

STAGE 2: By this stage, the kidneys will have deteriorated further and the patient's GFR levels will be outside of the normal levels for those without kidney disease. Doctors will now determine how quickly the disease is progressing. Guidance regarding blood pressure and sugar consumption will likely remain the same as at stage 1, and doctor visits should occur more frequently to monitor symptoms.

STAGE 3: GFR levels will have dropped significantly and at this stage doctors will start by checking for signs of additional complications including bone disease and anemia so that these can be treated accordingly. Monitoring check-ups will take place extremely frequently, if not daily.

STAGE 4: By this point, kidney function will have deteriorated further and GFR levels will have dropped dramatically. Doctors will very closely monitor the patient for potentially life-threatening complications, and the available options (should the kidneys fail completely) are discussed and determined with the patient.

STAGE 5: Those with stage 5 kidney disease have an extremely low GFR level and will be experiencing kidney failure. Dialysis or a kidney transplant are the options for somebody with stage 5 kidney disease. At this point, palliative care will likely be offered, depending on the pain, symptoms and side effects of the treatment given.

II
DIETARY CHOICES FOR A HEALTHIER LIFESTYLE

Your dietary and lifestyle choices can make a huge difference to your daily life, the symptoms you experience and in the early stages of kidney disease, the rate at which this develops. Changes can even prevent your kidneys from deteriorating, give you more energy, help you maintain a healthy weight, and prevent illnesses and infections. Overall there are four main elements that you should be focusing on within your diet: phosphorous, potassium, sodium and protein intake should be limited and by making these changes in the early stages of the disease, you may even be able to prevent a far stricter diet in the later stages of the disease.

Unfortunately, the diet many of us consume in the US and other western countries is not beneficial to our health. What nutritionists have termed the 'Standard American Diet' is unhealthy in many different respects: whilst including high levels of saturated fats, processed foods and animal fats, it is also light on complex carbohydrates, fiber, fruits and vegetables. All of this leads to a dramatically increased chance of stroke, heart disease, obesity, cancer and of course, kidney disease.

One of the main issues in this diet is the processed food, which is when chemicals have been added to food in order to preserve and make readily available to the consumer. In addition to these chemicals, processed foods include upwards of four times as much sugar as their natural counterparts. Excessive sugar levels increase the risk of type 2 diabetes, raises cholesterol levels, and creates a build-up of fat around the liver. As the liver works alongside the kidneys to remove toxins from the body, it is clear how these dietary choices can drastically increase the risk of kidney disease. It is always best to consult your doctor and nutritionist to devise a meal plan specifically suited to your needs and the stage of the disease you are in. It is also important that you monitor and control your calorie intake as a loss of appetite is commonly experienced as a side effect of the disease and therefore weight loss needs to be carefully monitored.

HEALTHY DIETARY CHOICES

This section will cover the choices you can make to ensure a healthy diet and the best treatment for your kidneys. Advice and guidance will differ according to what stage of the disease you're in, however, the principles remain similar throughout. Check with your doctor or nutritionist to ensure your diet plans are the best for you. Healthy food types and recommendations are outlined as well as food types and groups to consider avoiding or cutting down.

CARBOHYDRATES AND FIBER: Although carbohydrates may be difficult to process at later stages of kidney disease, they provide a vital source of energy that can combat the feelings of lethargy. As a low protein diet is recommended, carbohydrates can also help to replace calories. Some carbohydrates are also sources of fiber. It is recommended that you eat at least 25 grams of fiber per day, even when suffering from stage 5 kidney disease and undergoing dialysis. You may become frustrated when trying to count your fiber levels as many high fibrous foods are also high in potassium, phosphorous and fluid (all of which are restricted). The food lists in chapter three are a useful starting point for ingredients and their various nutritional values.

FATS: Fats often get a bad reputation as we don't often distinguish between healthy and unhealthy fats. Polyunsaturated and monounsaturated fats are healthy when consumed in moderation, whereas transfats and saturated fats should be avoided.

If you need to consume extra calories because of weight loss, these 'good' types of fat are great as part of a balanced diet. Too much fat, particularly transfats, can lead to a rapid increase in cholesterol, worsening symptoms experienced and also increasing your risk of heart disease. This is in turn linked to diabetes and high blood pressure, so it is always advised that you consume healthy fats in moderation and steer clear of the unhealthy fats altogether if possible. Oily fishes like tuna, salmon, and mackerel are excellent sources of these good fats. Choose oils for cooking and dressing such as coconut oil, canola oil, and olive oil, instead of sesame and vegetable oils.

PROTEIN: Although bodybuilders usually come to mind when we think of protein, it is actually an essential component of our diets and vital for repairing tissues, keeping infections at bay, and of course building muscle, even in the most exercise-phobic of us! If you have chronic kidney disease in the first few stages, it is still usually advised to consume protein for up to 15% of your daily diet, with carbohydrates and fats making up 85%. This is the same amount recommended for an average adult's daily intake. At stage 4 this recommendation usually decreases to only 10% protein. During stage 5, and if you are on dialysis, the dialysis will filter out the waste toxins from your body as well as protein, therefore it is crucial for you to include protein as part of your diet. Please note that you must follow your doctor's advice on how much protein you should be consuming at each stage, as it depends on various factors such as your height, weight and which stage of the disease you have. Always consult a professional for individual guidance before making any changes to your diet.

PHOSPHORUS AND CALCIUM: Phosphates are salt compounds which include salt as well as other minerals; they work, as does calcium, to strengthen and keep our bones healthy. Extra phosphorous in the blood is usually removed by our kidneys, but kidney disease will prevent this process from functioning as it should. Unfortunately, it's not as simple as just removing all phosphates from your diet as they are pretty much in most foods, but we can look out for those high in phosphorous. Chapter Three provides a list of foods and identifies whether they are low, medium or high in phosphorous. You should typically stay away from processed foods as these often contain additives. Too much phosphorus can also lead to a calcium deficit which can, in turn, lead to the extreme bouts of itchiness that many chronic kidney disease sufferers report. If low calcium levels persist this can lead to further pain, a general weakening of the bones, and even bone disease. Your doctor may recommend taking a calcium supplement if your phosphorus levels remain too high. After this, medicines known as phosphorous binders may be required but always consult a professional.

FLUIDS: As the kidneys start to decrease in functionality, waste toxins and excess liquids are not removed from the body as they should be. This may lead to your doctor recommending you limit the liquids you consume. Foods with high liquid content also need to be considered as well as the drinks you consume, for instance, fruits such as apples and pears, milk, soups, ice creams etc. This is more likely during the later stages of kidney disease and you should consult a professional for specific advice.

POTASSIUM: A mineral that plays an essential role in keeping your heart healthy as well as regulating water levels in the body. Again, this is another mineral that is usually removed when in excess through the kidney filtration system. Too much of one particular mineral is problematic as the kidneys just cannot remove it in the way they can when they are completely healthy. That being said, extremely low levels of potassium are also harmful and kidney disease sufferers may experience either extreme. This is unique to you so will need to be monitored by a professional. Potassium is commonly found in many fruits and vegetables - stick with watermelon, tangerines, pineapple, berries, apples, cherries, pears, grapes, and peaches as low potassium fruits.

IRON: Anyone whose chronic kidney disease has resulted in anemia will need extra iron in their diet. Options that are high in iron include iron-fortified cereals, kidney beans, lima beans, chicken, pork, beef, and liver. As some iron-rich sources may conflict with other dietary considerations such as protein, ensure you find out from your doctor which sources of iron you can have.

STAGE SPECIFIC ADVICE

Your dietary needs and requirements will continue to change throughout the stages of kidney disease. The following information will give you a general idea of the key dietary considerations and guidance but please always consult a healthcare professional before making changes to your diet.

STAGE 1 AND STAGE 2: These stages are typically combined together because at this point the kidneys are still working at a similar level to healthy kidneys and symptoms may not be experienced yet. It is essential however at this stage to preserve as much of the kidneys' proper functioning as possible. This list below gives guidance on a variety of dietary choices that are usually recommended during these stages of the disease:

- Reduce dairy consumption in order to better control your protein intake.
- Increase your fiber intake by consuming more cereal, vegetables and fruits.
- Eat more seafood and poultry than red meat.
- Baking, shallow frying in healthy oils, and steaming are better methods for cooking than deep frying.
- A maximum of 6oz. meat is recommended each day.
- Cut down or avoid processed foods completely.
- Keep alcohol consumption to a minimum i.e. 1-2 glasses per week or none at all.
- Consume the recommended amount of calories for your height, gender and activity levels.
- Use herbs and spices and balsamic vinegar to season your salads, vegetables and foods instead of salts and shop-bought salad dressings (usually high in preservatives and fats).
- Sodium: 1-200mg. per day.
- Potassium: 2-4000mg. per day.
- Phosphorous - 800-1200mg. per day depending on weight.
- Protein - 0.8-1.2g per kilo of body weight.

STAGE 3: Primary goals in this stage include managing levels of minerals and vitamins, hormones, fat cells, lipids, and glucose. While some will need to focus on losing weight, others may need to gain weight due to anemia or a loss of appetite. A dietitian or doctor should determine the number of calories you should be consuming each day.

- Limit or avoid trans and saturated fats. Replace with monounsaturated and polyunsaturated fats.
- Fluid retention is not typically monitored during stage three, nevertheless, it is important to be aware of sudden swelling, weight gain, blood pressure spikes or urination issues as they can all indicate a decrease in the kidneys' ability to expel water.
- Vitamin D supplements may be recommended if you need to lower your phosphorous levels.
- Sodium: 1200-2000mg. per day.
- Potassium: 2-4000mg. per day.
- Phosphorous - 1-1200mg. per day depending on weight.
- Protein - 0.6-0.8g per kilo of body weight.

STAGE 4: The quality of kidney functions will have been dramatically decreased at this point which is likely to lead to issues such as fluid retention, fatigue, trouble focusing, sleep difficulty, nerve issues, bad breath, abnormal tastes, loss of appetite, vomiting, and nausea.

- Closely monitor and control potassium, phosphorous and sodium intake. The guidance will be specific to your needs and should come from a healthcare professional.
- Fluid retention varies from person to person during stage 4 depending on how well the kidneys are still working. Some type of fluid retention is almost always present, which is why it is important to monitor your fluid intake carefully.
- Sodium: 1-2000mg. per day.
- Potassium: 2-4000mg. per day.
- Phosphorous - 750-1000mg. per day depending on weight.
- Protein - 20-30g max. per day depending on dialysis treatment and weight.

STAGE 5: Many factors need to be taken into consideration at this stage when it comes to diet including response to dialysis, the likelihood of a transplant, your current nutritional concerns, and your latest results from medical tests. Uremia during this stage makes it difficult for many people to eat regularly, which in turn brings on additional dietary concerns in terms of malnutrition.

- During stage 5 it is important to ensure that you are still consuming the recommended amount of vegetables, fruits and grains. Wholegrains and those high in potassium or sodium are to be avoided altogether.
- Cholesterol and saturated fats need to be cut out almost completely.
- Sodium intake will be extremely restricted at this point to help monitor fluid consumption.
- Calcium levels will be watched closely at this point as some people continue to need supplements while levels in others may return to normal (in which case calcium supplementation must be stopped).
- The amount of protein advised will likely be increased to counteract the effects of dialysis.
- Vitamin supplements for B, C, D, and iron will all most likely be added to the diet to supplement the dialysis.
- Sodium: 1-2000mg. per day.
- Potassium: 2-2500mg. per day.
- Phosphorous - 7mg. per kilo of body weight.
- Protein -20-30g max. per day.

III

EATING OUT AND SHOPPING GUIDE

It is a lot easier to stick to a healthy diet if you make the right choices on your grocery shops; keep the kitchen stocked with an array of healthy ingredients and you won't find yourself calling the takeaway or grabbing something on the go. That being said, eating out can be quite daunting. You don't want to miss out on spending time with your loved ones and doing the things you enjoy, but you worry about temptation or possibly causing a scene. This chapter will help you make the right decisions about what to keep in your kitchen as well as provide you with hints and tips on what to choose when you're out and about. Additionally, it is important to always read the labels and monitor the levels of potassium, sodium, phosphorous, protein and fats according to your needs.

KIDNEY SUPER FOODS

The following tables list a variety of food types and their dietary specifics. It is important to note that these are based on the given serving sizes and therefore, increasing the serving size will increase the levels of phosphorous, sodium etc. Stick to these serving sizes as one serving.

L= LOW
(Potassium - Less than 150mg/serving, Phosphorous - Less than 150mg/serving, Protein - Less than 10g per serving, Sodium - less than 150mg per serving)

M = MEDIUM
(Potassium - 151 -250mg/serving, Phosphorous - 151- 250mg/serving, Protein -10 - 20g per serving, Sodium - 150 - 250mg per serving)

H = HIGH
(Potassium - More than 251mg/serving, Phosphorous - More than 251mg/serving, Protein -More than 20g per serving, Sodium - More than 251mg per serving)

Fruits 1/2 cup	Fiber	Potassium	Phosphorous	Protein	Sodium
raspberries	H	L	L	L	L
blackberries	H	M	L	L	L
pears	H	M	L	L	L
apples cooked	H	L	L	L	L
apples raw	H	M	L	L	L
tangerine	H	M	L	L	L

Fruits 1/2 cup	Fiber	Potassium	Phosphorous	Protein	Sodium
strawberries	H	M	L	L	L
apricots	H	M = 1 apricot	L	L	L
blackberries	H	M	L	L	L
blueberries	H	L	L	L	L
lemons & limes		L	L	L	L
dried cranberries and cranberry juice	H	L	L	L	L
grapes	H	L	L	L	L
raw fig	H	L	L	L	L
grapefruit	H	M	L	L	L
plums	H	L	L	L	L
pineapple	H	L	L	L	L
raspberries	H	L	L	L	L

Vegetables 1/2 cup	Fiber	Potassium	Phosphorous	Protein	Sodium
peas	H	M	L	L	L
beans (green)	H	L	L	L	L
carrots	H	L	L	L	L
asparagus	H	M	L	L	L
cauliflower	H	L	L	L	L
cabbage (boiled)	H	L	L	L	L
broccoli	H	M	L	L	L
corn	H	M	L	L	L
eggplant	H	M	L	L	L
okra cooked	H	L	L	L	L
chickpeas	H	M	M	L	L
leek	H	M	L	L	L
cucumber	L	L	L	L	L
lettuce	L	L	M	L	L
onions raw	H	L	L	L	L
radishes	L	L	L	L	L
spinach raw	L	L	M	L	L
garlic	H	H	M	L	L
red bell peppers	H	L	L	L	L

Grains and other 1/2 cup	Fiber	Potassium	Phosphorous	Protein	Sodium
flaxseed	H	L	H	M	L
barley	H	L	L	L	L
brown rice	H	L	M	L	L
cornflakes	H	L	L	L	L
corn grits	H	L	L	L	H
oatmeal	H	L	M	L	L
unsweetened cocoa 2 tbsp	L	L	L	L	L
wholewheat bread 2 slices	H	L	M	L	L
soy milk	L	M	L	L	L
pasta	H	L	L	L	L
tofu	H	M	L	M	L
1 rice cake	L	L	L	L	L
unsalted -almonds, cashews, hazelnuts, pine nuts, pistachios, walnuts, peanuts	H	H	H	H	L

Grains and other 1/2 cup	Fiber	Potassium	Phosphorous	Protein	Sodium
lentils, white beans, soy-beans	H	H	M	M	L
wholegrain flour	H	L	L	H	L

Meat and fish 3 oz Dairy 1/2 cup	Fiber	Potassium	Phosphorous	Protein	Sodium
feta cheese	L	L	L	M	H
brie cheese	L	L	L	H	H
duck	L	L	L	H	L
wholewheat bread 2 slices	H	L	M	L	L
chicken/turkey breast	L	L	M	H	L
beef - ground, sirloin, chuck	L	L	M	H	L
egg x 1	L	L	L	H	L

Meat and fish 3 oz Dairy 1/2 cup	Fiber	Potassium	Phosphorous	Protein	Sodium
shrimp	L	L	L	H	H
cod/halibut/ pollock/salmon	L	L	H	H	L
pork leg/chops	L	H	M	H	L
tuna, canned or yellowfin	L	L	H	H	M
greek/plain yogurt	L	L	M	H	L
milk skimmed	L	M	L	H	L
cottage cheese	L	L	M	H	H

THE SUPER FOODS SUMMED UP!

This section outlines some of the top super foods that you may want to consider incorporating into your diet. Depending on the stage of kidney disease you are at, certain foods may not be suitable for you. Please always check with your doctor or dietitian before adding or removing foods from your diet.

RED BELL PEPPERS: Red bell peppers are ideal for those suffering from chronic kidney disease as they are full of fiber, folic acid, vitamin B6, vitamin C and vitamin A while also being low in potassium. Another benefit for the kidneys is the high concentration of lycopene - an antioxidant that will increase kidney performance. Red bell peppers taste great in chicken or tuna salads or simply eaten with a low sodium dip. Roasted, they make a great addition to any salad or sandwich. They also add a mild kick to kebabs, egg dishes or as a part of a ground turkey or beef meal.

CABBAGE: Cabbage contains high amounts of phytochemicals which break down toxins, improve cardiovascular health and fight cancer. What's more, cabbage is a great source of folic acid, B6, fiber, vitamin C and vitamin K while still being low in potassium. Cabbage is a great addition to fish tacos or coleslaw and can be microwaved, steamed or boiled depending.

CAULIFLOWER: Cauliflower contains numerous compounds that help the liver to remove toxins from the body; it is high in fiber, folate, and vitamin C. Cauliflower is delicious with a simple dip, in salads, boiled or steamed. Cauliflower can be a great substitute for things like rice and potatoes and can be flavored using herbs, spices, and mustard.

GARLIC: Garlic is great used to replace salt for flavoring and seasoning and it also naturally lowers cholesterol and mitigates inflation. Garlic has fewer anti-inflammatory and anti-clotting effects once it has been cooked so is best consumed raw for maximum results.

ONION: Raw onions are low in potassium and high in chromium which is beneficial when it comes to helping the metabolism maintain its proper function. They can be consumed cooked or raw.

APPLES: High in fiber and vitamin content which helps to mitigate inflammation, apples have been linked to decreasing cancer risk, preventing heart disease, easing constipation and lowering cholesterol. They are just as healthy cooked as raw, and can also be consumed as a juice. Those who have been advised to restrict their water intake should avoid apples because of their significant water content.

CRANBERRIES: Cranberries are very acidic and help to prevent harmful bacteria from forming in the bladder, thus preventing infections in the urinary tract. They are also vitamin rich which can help to reduce the risk of heart disease or cancer. Cranberries are just as healthy when dried as they are when fresh and can be added to most salads or cereals for a delicious twist. Cranberry juice should be avoided for those on a restricted liquid intake.

BLUEBERRIES: High in antioxidants, fiber and vitamin C, blueberries also help to mitigate inflammation. Their manganese content helps prevent bone related issues that may occur as a result of a calcium deficiency. Blueberries can be eaten raw, dried, baked, in a smoothie, or with cereal.

RASPBERRIES: Also high in antioxidants, these little superfoods are known to help reduce cancer cells or tumor growth.

STRAWBERRIES: High in fiber, manganese, vitamin C and other vitamins and minerals which are known to help prevent cancer, maintain heart health and mitigate inflammation.

CHERRIES: Eating cherries daily has been shown to measurably reduce the amount of inflammation that those experiencing chronic kidney disease experience. They are also high in antioxidants as well as phytochemicals which help reduce the risk of heart disease. Cherries are great on their own, in desserts and also as a sauce for either pork or lamb.

RED GRAPES: Red grapes get their color from flavonoids which help to maintain heart health, reduce the risk of blood clots and improve oxidation and overall blood flow. They are also known to help reduce the risk of cancer and ease inflammation. Choose grapes the most vibrant in color. Frozen grapes taste delicious and are also thirst quenching, which is great if you are having to control your water intake.

EGG WHITES: Egg whites are pure protein; they are also lower in phosphorus than egg yolks, and they contain a wealth of vital amino acids. Egg whites can be eaten on their own, in salads, with tuna, or even in smoothies for those not on a liquid restricted diet.

FISH: Besides being a great source of protein, fish is known to be an anti-inflammatory agent thanks to its omega-3 content. Additional fats found in fish can help reduce the risk of heart disease as well as cancer. The healthiest fish in terms of omega-3 content are rainbow trout, herring, mackerel, tuna, albacore, and salmon.

OLIVE OIL: Olive oil has been linked to a reduced risk of both heart disease and cancer. Extra virgin olive oil contains higher levels of antioxidants than regular olive oil, making it a great choice for cooking, as a dip, marinade or dressing.

KALE: Loaded with flavonoids and carotenoids, both of which can reduce the risk of heart disease and cancer, kale is also full of calcium, vitamin C, vitamin A and vitamin K. Kale is a great snack choice as it can be baked and consumed as a chip.

VITAMINS & SUPPLEMENTS: Vitamins and supplements that you would usually buy in shops should be avoided when on a renal diet as they may contain high levels that cannot be regulated by the kidneys anymore. Your healthcare professional may prescribe you a vitamin suitable for kidney disease patients, so please consult with them first.

FOODS TO AVOID OR CUT DOWN

DAIRY: It is sometimes advised to limit your consumption of dairy whilst on a renal diet, this will help monitor your protein intake as well as control the amount of fat you eat. Try swapping full-fat cheddar and parmesan for cottage cheese or brie.

CAFFEINE: Caffeine is a stimulant which is hard for the kidneys to filter. Moreover, consuming caffeine on an empty stomach has been linked to the formation of kidney stones and can also lead to an increase in calcium levels found in the urine. Try reducing the amount of caffeine you drink slowly; this will prevent withdrawal symptoms and ensure healthier functioning kidneys for longer. Green tea is a great caffeine-free alternative to coffee and tea but it boosts energy in the same way as caffeine does, making you feel great.

ARTIFICIAL SWEETENER: Avoid artificial sweeteners like saccharin and opt for Stevia if you need something to sweeten up your teas or meals.

SODA: Soda is harmful to both your kidneys as well as your bones, in fact, drinking just 32 oz. of soda per day is known to measurably increase your risk of chronic kidney disease. Avoid soda on a kidney-friendly diet.

GMO's: Genetically modified organisms are likely to increase the number of free radicals present in foods; the chemicals and toxins in these foods cannot be filtered by the kidneys properly.

POTATOES: Sweet potatoes and white potatoes are high in potassium and should be monitored. They can be leached by soaking them in warm water or boiling twice prior to cooking to remove excess potassium. Sweet potatoes come with many other vitamins and minerals so it is important to consult your doctor or dietitian to find out whether you can include potatoes in your diet and what quantities.

TOMATOES: Tomatoes are also high in potassium. Canned tomatoes with no added salt or sugar can be consumed in moderation. Please consult your doctor or dietitian to find out whether you need to avoid tomatoes completely.

TIPS FOR EATING OUT:

Firstly, don't be embarrassed to make specific requests when eating out. Your health is more important than seeming to make a fuss and most of the time servers will be more than happy to meet your needs. If not, they're not worth your custom!

- Always ask for vegetables and side salads to be served plain and cooked dry without oil or butter.
- Avoid deep-fried and breadcrumbed foods as these are often cooked in huge quantities of bad oils.
- When choosing steak, ask or opt for a smaller cut and have sides of vegetables, salads or suitable grains to fill you up.
- Seafood, chicken, and turkey are better options but ensure they're baked, poached, steamed or boiled. If shallow fried, ask for them to cook this in olive oil.
- Try smaller or half portions if you're going to have a starter and a main.
- Ask for olive oils or vinegar on the side so you can control the amount you put on your food.
- Limit your alcohol intake and order a small glass. Ask waiters and waitresses not to top this up if you're somewhere fancy!
- Print the list of foods above or perhaps keep it electronically on your phone so you can easily check food types and opt for the best choice when dining out.
- If visiting friends and family members, share this list with them so they can make the best choices for everyone and not worry about whether they are doing the right thing.

IV

COOKING TIPS

Hopefully, by now, you know more about the symptoms, causes, and stages of kidney disease. You also know a little more about kidney-friendly foods as well as foods you should potentially limit or avoid. This chapter outlines the best cooking methods for a healthy diet, which is in line with healthy eating advice in general. It also provides ways of combating sodium and potassium.

COMBATING SODIUM:

Salt is often overused to season our foods and act as preservatives in packaged foods. In fact, taste tests show that as little as one-eighth of a teaspoon is enough for most people to notice. Reduce the amount of salt you add to foods gradually and always check the labels of ingredients for their sodium levels.

If using canned vegetables, ensure the juice or broth has no added salt by checking the labels; fresh vegetables are always a better option. You can easily make broths and soups out of leftover vegetables or bones from chicken, turkey and even beef. A chicken stock recipe is included in the poultry section. Herbs and spices, as well as balsamic or white vinegar, can be used to replace salt when cooking or dressing foods. Sometimes, something sweet can be used for a surprising twist on your favorite meal, for example, a squeeze of fresh lime or lemon juice. Likewise, different cooking methods result in a variety of flavors from the same ingredients! Experiment with baking and roasting as well as grilling to liven up the same foods in the kitchen.

COMBATING POTASSIUM:

Boiling vegetables helps reduce potassium; if you've got extra time or you're really prepared, soaking them in warm water for a few hours helps this process. Cleaning and peeling potatoes and boiling twice is sufficient enough for stripping excess potassium out of the potatoes. When making stews and soups it is better to boil the vegetables first so as not to allow potassium to soak into the rest of the pot. If cooking with frozen or canned vegetables, they should be rinsed and soaked prior to use in order to reduce potassium levels. Low-sodium labelled products are not the ideal choice as these often contain other chemicals that are harmful to the body. Instead, use the methods described above to reduce potassium as much as possible and try using ingredients with a low potassium content where you can.

VI
GETTING STARTED

CONSIDER YOUR LIFESTYLE

Follows the tips below to make the transition to a healthy, kidney friendly diet as easy as possible.

- Eat a large breakfast, a medium-sized lunch, and a small dinner.
- Increase consumption of vegetables and fruits daily.
- Switch to olive oil based dressings.
- Try healthy snacks instead of quick and processed snacks e.g. roasted kale chips, plain yogurt, fruits and nuts in moderation.
- Eating smaller meals with a healthy snack in between will work for those needing to control calorie intake as well as those who have lost their appetite.
- Stay away from juices and sodas as they both contain high amounts of processed ingredients and sugar.
- Drink fresh water and green teas, but be aware of how much liquid you should be consuming each day.
- Don't eat after 8 pm to allow your body and kidneys time to function before sleep.
- Find an activity or hobby to prevent boredom eating.
- Get into the habit of reading labels on foods and looking for sodium, potassium, phosphorous, protein and calorie amounts.
- Eat a balanced diet to include protein, healthy fats and carbohydrates according to your diagnosis and personal needs.
- Stop smoking.
- Stay positive by asking friends and family members to try the healthy eating with you.
- If you have a bad day, don't let it throw you off for good.
- Log your symptoms as well as what you eat in a journal every day. This will help you keep track not only of how much and what types of foods you've eaten but also how they make you feel.
- Keep up with scheduled appointments and monitor your blood pressure to ensure it is not too high.
- If you're diabetic, ensure you monitor your condition and consult your doctor about specific sugar recommendations.
- Seek professional advice early as well as the support from loved ones. This can be an incredibly emotional time and you shouldn't have to experience it alone. Therapy might even be an option if you wish to talk about your feelings to a third party.

EXERCISE

The level of exercise you can safely perform while dealing with your chronic kidney disease will vary greatly depending on your current prognosis, the symptoms you are showing and your general level of physical fitness. Exercise is known to be especially helpful in the early stages of the disease and can help to fight off the initial feelings of fatigue that many people experience.

Exercise is useful for those who are looking to lose weight as a way to help mitigate numerous conditions that can lead to chronic kidney failure. Exercise can also strengthen the heart and is also known to help with anxiety as well as depression.

For those who have to limit their fluid intake, strenuous exercise is not advised as you will become dehydrated and need to consume higher quantities of water. In this case yoga and light walks are advised to keep fit and healthy whilst not exerting yourself too much. Speak with your healthcare professional for specific guidance.

BEFORE YOU GET STARTED

Chronic kidney disease is a life-changing diagnosis. However, there are ways of living with the disease whilst maintaining a healthy life. The following recipes have all been created to help you to continue enjoying delicious, healthy meals.

Each recipe is listed with its key nutritional values. It is crucial that you follow your doctor's professional guidance for your daily dietary intake; this will be unique to each individual and depends on various factors. Please note that each recipe contains different amounts of protein, sodium, phosphorous and potassium so you will need to plan and track each meal in order to stay within your daily limits.

Happy cooking!

BREAKFAST

TURKEY AND SPINACH SCRAMBLE ON MELBA TOAST

SERVES 4 / PREP TIME: 3 MINUTES / COOK TIME: 15 MINUTES

No need to add eggs, this scramble is an iron and protein rich start to the day.

1 TSP EXTRA VIRGIN OLIVE OIL

1 CUP COOKED AND DICED TURKEY BREAST

1 CUP RAW SPINACH

1/2 GARLIC CLOVE, MINCED

1 TSP NUTMEG, GRATED OR DRIED

4 SLICES MELBA TOAST

1 TSP BALSAMIC VINEGAR

1. Heat a skillet on a medium heat and add oil.
2. Add your turkey pieces to the pan and heat through thoroughly for 6-8 minutes.
3. Now add the spinach, garlic, and nutmeg and allow to cook for a further 6 minutes, stirring every now and then to prevent the garlic from browning.
4. Plate up the Melba toast and top with the spinach and turkey scramble.
5. Drizzle with a little balsamic vinegar if desired and serve.

Per serving: Calories: 88; Fat: 2g; Carbohydrates: 5g; Phosphorus: 102mg ; Potassium: 170mg; Sodium: 56mg; Protein: 12g

MEXICAN STYLE BURRITOS

SERVES 2 / PREP TIME: 5 MINUTES / COOK TIME: 15 MINUTES

This simple poached egg dish is a great way to turn up the heat for breakfast. Just add salsa. Skip the eggs if you have been advised to cut egg yolks from your diet.

---

2 WHITE TORTILLAS

1 TBSP CANOLA OIL

1/4 CUP RED ONION, DICED

1/2 RED CHILI, DE-SEEDED AND FINELY CHOPPED

1/4 CUP RED BELL PEPPERS, DICED

2 EGGS

1 TBSP CILANTRO, FINELY CHOPPED

1 LIME, FRESHLY SQUEEZED

---

1. Turn the broiler to a medium heat and place the tortillas underneath for 1-2 minutes on each side or until lightly toasted. Place to one side but keep broiler on.
2. Now heat the oil in a skillet over a medium heat and sauté the onion, chili and bell peppers for 5-6 minutes until soft.
3. Crack the eggs over the top of the onions and peppers and place skillet under the broiler for 5-6 minutes or until the eggs are cooked.
4. Serve half the eggs and vegetables on top of each tortilla and sprinkle with cilantro and lime juice to serve.

Per serving: Calories: 197; Fat: 12g; Carbohydrates: 17g; Phosphorus: 178mg; Potassium: 208mg; Sodium: 201g; Protein: 7g

BAKED EGG MUFFINS

SERVES 6 / PREP TIME: 15 MINUTES / COOK TIME: 25 MINUTES

So easy to prepare - these make delicious breakfasts or snacks between meals. Please consult your doctor or dietitian to find out if you can still include whole eggs in your diet before preparing this recipe.

1/3 CUP ONION, DICED

1/3 CUP MUSHROOMS, DICED

1/3 CUP BELL PEPPER, DICED

1/2 CUP COOKED SKINLESS TURKEY OR CHICKEN PIECES

6 LARGE EGGS

1 TSP DRIED THYME

1. Line a muffin pan with 6 wrappers.
2. Mix vegetables together in a separate bowl.
3. Next, spoon the vegetable mixture and turkey pieces into the muffin trays up to about 2/3 full, allowing room for the eggs.
4. Beat the eggs with the thyme in a separate bowl or jug.
5. Pour beaten eggs into each muffin tray - leave 1cm gap at the top.
6. Place the muffin tray in the oven and bake for approximately 25 minutes or until eggs are cooked through.
7. Remove egg muffins and serve.

Per serving: Calories: 101; Fat: 5g; Carbohydrates: 3g; Phosphorus: 141mg; Potassium: 173mg; Sodium: 222mg; Protein: 11g

SPRING GREEN OMELET

SERVES 2 / PREP TIME: 5 MINUTES / COOK TIME: 15 MINUTES

A light and fresh breakfast, made with your favorite vegetables. Use just the egg whites if your doctor has advised you to cut egg yolks from your diet.

1 TBSP EXTRA VIRGIN OLIVE OIL	1 LARGE EGG
1/2 LEEK, DICED	2 LARGE EGG WHITES
1/3 CUP ZUCCHINI, DICED	PINCH OF BLACK PEPPER
1 GREEN ONION, DICED	2 TBSP WATER

1. Heat olive oil in a skillet over a medium to high heat.
2. Sauté the vegetables for 4-5 minutes.
3. Using a whisk, mix together the egg, egg whites, pepper, and water in a separate bowl.
4. Pour the eggs over the vegetables in the skillet and cook for 5-6 minutes until the edges begin to set.
5. Use a spatula to gently lift the edges of the omelet and turn over in the pan.
6. Fold the omelet in half and continue cooking for 3-4 minutes.
7. Remove omelet from the pan and cut in half to serve.

Per serving: Calories: 129; Fat: 9g; Carbohydrates: 5g; Phosphorus: 71mg; Potassium: 171mg; Sodium: 218mg; Protein: 7g

SWEET PANCAKES

SERVES 5 / PREP TIME: 10 MINUTES / COOK TIME: 5 MINUTES

A mouthwatering breakfast!

---

1 CUP ALL-PURPOSE FLOUR

1 TBSP GRANULATED SUGAR

2 TSP BAKING POWDER

2 LARGE EGG WHITES

1 CUP 1% LOW-FAT MILK/ALMOND

2 TBSP CANOLA OIL

1 TBSP MAPLE EXTRACT

---

1. In a bowl mix the flour, sugar, and baking powder.
2. Make a well in the center and place to one side.
3. In a larger bowl mix the egg whites, milk, oil and maple extract.
4. Add the egg mixture to the well and gently mix outwards until a batter is formed.
5. Heat a skillet over a medium heat.
6. Add 1/5 of the batter to the pan and cook for about 2 minutes on each side or until the pancake is golden.
7. Use a spatula to flip the pancake halfway through.
8. Repeat with the remaining batter.
9. Serve warm.

Per serving: Calories: 187; Fat: 6g; Carbohydrates: 27g; Phosphorus: 116mg; Potassium: 130mg; Sodium: 260mg; Protein: 6g

RAINBOW VEGGIE FRITTATA

SERVES 4 / PREP TIME: 5 MINUTES / COOK TIME: 30 MINUTES

Yellow squash is lower in potassium than potatoes and tastes scrumptious with the zucchini in this breakfast treat. Use just the egg whites if your doctor has advised you to cut egg yolks from your diet.

---

2 TBSP COCONUT OR EXTRA VIRGIN OLIVE OIL

1 YELLOW SQUASH, PEELED, SLICED AND BOILED TO REMOVE EXCESS POTASSIUM

2 ZUCCHINIS, PEELED, SLICED AND SOAKED IN WARM WATER

5 EGGS

2 TSP PARSLEY

1 TSP CRACKED BLACK PEPPER

---

1. Heat the oil in a skillet under a broiler on a medium heat.
2. Spread the squash slices across the skillet and cook for 5 minutes.
3. Add the zucchini to the skillet and cook for a further 5 minutes.
4. Meanwhile, whisk the eggs and parsley in a separate bowl, and season with black pepper to taste before pouring over the veggies in the skillet.
5. Cook for 10 minutes on a low heat until golden brown.
6. Plate up and serve into 4 portions. Try with a side salad for a lovely brunch idea.

Per serving: Calories: 184; Fat: 13g; Carbohydrates: 11g; Phosphorus: 198mg; Potassium: 385mg; Sodium: 239mg; Protein: 9g

LEMON AND BERRY CREPES

SERVES 4 / PREP TIME: 1 HOUR / COOK TIME: 15 MINUTES

So much healthier than the pre-packaged or restaurant versions but just as delicious! Please consult your doctor or dietitian to find out if you can still include whole eggs in your diet before preparing this recipe.

3 LARGE EGGS

1-1/3 CUPS ALMOND MILK

3/4 CUP WHITE FLOUR

1 TSP COCONUT OIL

1 CUP FRESH OR FROZEN BLUEBERRIES,

BLACKBERRIES AND RASPBERRIES TO SERVE

1 LEMON

1. Whisk eggs and milk together.
2. Slowly sift flour in and continue mixing for 1 minute.
3. Cover and let sit for 1 hour.
4. Pour batter into a bowl.
5. Heat an 8-inch crepe pan or skillet over a medium-high heat.
6. Drizzle with coconut oil.
7. Pour the batter into the skillet in 1/4 cup servings.
8. Make sure the batter lies evenly, twirling the pan to form a crepe or pancake shape.
9. Cook for 3-4 minutes until edges are slightly brown and you can use your spatula to lift the edges without it sticking.
10. Turn the crepe and cook for 1 minute on the other side.
11. Remove from pan and place on serving plate.
12. Top with fresh fruits and a squeeze of lemon juice and roll to serve.

Per serving: Calories: 184; Fat: 4g; Carbohydrates: 30g; Phosphorus: 102mg; Potassium: 156mg; Sodium: 177mg; Protein: 7g

DELICIOUS FRENCH TOAST

SERVES 4 / PREP TIME: 5 MINUTES   COOK TIME: 10 MINUTES

A popular breakfast treat that you can continue to enjoy! Use just the egg whites if your doctor has advised you to cut egg yolks from your diet.

4 SLICES LOW-SODIUM WHITE BREAD, 3/4" THICK

3 LARGE EGGS

1 1/4 CUP UNSWEETENED ALMOND MILK

2 TBSP CANOLA OIL

1. Trim the crusts and slice the bread diagonally.
2. Lightly beat the eggs and add to the almond milk.
3. Pour oil into a skillet and heat over a medium heat.
4. Dip the bread into the egg mixture and add to the skillet for 3-4 minutes each side or until lightly brown.

Per serving: Calories: 212; Fat: 12g; Carbohydrates: 18g; Phosphorus: 104mg; Potassium: 121mg; Sodium: 287mg; Protein: 7g

BAKED CHERRY PANCAKES

SERVES 4 / PREP TIME: 5 MINUTES / COOK TIME: 30 MINUTES

A gluten-free dish, so simple to cook! Please consult your doctor or dietitian to find out if you can still include whole eggs in your diet before preparing this recipe.

---

2 TBSP COCONUT OIL

2 LARGE EGGS

1/2 CUP GLUTEN FREE WHITE FLOUR

1/2 CUP CHERRIES, FINELY CHOPPED

1/2 CUP RICE MILK (UNENRICHED)

---

1. Preheat the oven to 400°f/200°c/Gas Mark 6.
2. Add coconut oil to an oven proof skillet and place in oven until it has melted.
3. In a mixing bowl, whisk eggs until combined.
4. Add flour, cherries, and rice milk and mix until smooth.
5. Remove skillet from the oven and immediately pour the batter into the hot skillet.
6. Place back in oven and bake for 25 to 30 minutes until pancake has risen slightly and is golden brown in color.
7. Plate and cut into 4 portions to serve.
8. Top with extra fresh cherries to serve.

Per serving: Calories: 173; Fat: 9g; Carbohydrates: 18g; Phosphorus: 78mg; Potassium: 129mg; Sodium: 139mg; Protein: 5g

RHUBARB AND CUSTARD

A tasty fruity breakfast salad, rich in antioxidants. Please consult your doctor or dietitian to find out if you can still include whole eggs in your diet before preparing this recipe.

3 LARGE EGGS	PINCH OF CINNAMON
1 EGG YOLK	1 TBSP BROWN SUGAR
1 TSP VANILLA EXTRACT	1 RHUBARB PLANT, CHOPPED
2 CUPS ALMOND MILK	2 APPLES, CORED PEELED AND CHOPPED

1. Preheat the oven to 350°f/170°c/Gas Mark 4.
2. Add hot water to a deep baking tray (about 3/4 full) and place in oven.
3. In a large bowl, lightly beat all of the eggs and vanilla.
4. Heat a pan on a medium heat and add the almond milk, cinnamon, and brown sugar. Warm through but don't allow to boil.
5. Add the warm mixture to the eggs and mix.
6. Sieve the mixture into an oven dish.
7. Add the rhubarb and apple into the oven dish.
8. Add the oven dish to the baking tray so that it is sitting in the water (don't allow the water to overflow into the oven dish though!)
9. Bake for 35 minutes and serve warm.

Per serving: Calories: 174; Fat: 6g; Carbohydrates: 23g; Phosphorus: 119mg; Potassium: 353mg; Sodium: 258mg; Protein: 7g

FRUIT PUNCH PORRIDGE

SERVES 2 / PREP TIME: 5 MINUTES / COOK TIME: 20 MINUTES

Buckwheat is lower in potassium and phosphorous than oats and makes a tasty porridge.

---

2 CUPS WATER

1/2 CUP BUCKWHEAT

1 1/2 CUPS ALMOND MILK

1/4 GRAPEFRUIT, CHOPPED

1 TBSP HONEY

---

1. Bring the water to a boil on the stove, add the buckwheat and place the lid on the pan.
2. Lower heat slightly and allow to simmer for 7-10 minutes, checking to ensure water does not dry out.
3. When most of the water is absorbed, remove from the heat and allow to sit for 5 minutes.
4. Drain any excess water from the pan and stir in the almond milk, heating through for a further 5 minutes.
5. Now add the grapefruit and honey.
6. Serve warm!

Per serving: Calories: 228; Fat: 3g; Carbohydrates: 48g; Phosphorus: 106mg; Potassium: 243mg; Sodium: 131mg; Protein: 5g

POULTRY

HOMEMADE HEALTHY CHICKEN STOCK

SERVING SIZE: 1 CUP / PREP TIME: 10 MINUTES / COOK TIME: 4 HOURS

This homemade chicken stock is far healthier than shop bought and can be used in a lot of the recipes featured in this cookbook.

---

1 WHOLE ROASTING CHICKEN {AROUND 4-5LBS}

3 CARROTS, SOAKED IN WARM WATER

2 MEDIUM ONIONS

3 STALKS OF CELERY, SOAKED IN WARM WATER

4 GARLIC CLOVES, CRUSHED

2 BAY LEAVES

1 TBSP EACH DRIED ROSEMARY, THYME, PEPPER, TURMERIC

1 TBSP WHITE WINE VINEGAR

11-12 CUPS WATER

---

1. Rinse off your chicken and place in a large saucepan or soup pan (remove giblets but don't waste them; add them in to your stock bowl!)
2. Chop your vegetables into quarters (leave the skins on as they add to the taste and the nutrients) add to the pan.
3. Add the herbs, spices, pepper and vinegar to the pan.
4. Fill your pan with water so that the chicken and vegetables are completely covered.
5. Turn stove on high and bring to boiling point before reducing the heat and allowing the stock to simmer for 3-4 hours.
6. Check at intervals and top up with water if the ingredients become uncovered.
7. Take off the heat and carefully remove the chicken, placing to one side.
8. Strain the liquid from the stockpot into another bowl using a sieve.
9. Leave the stock and chicken to cool and place to one side.
10. Once cool, tear or cut the meat from the bones.
11. Add stock to a sealed container and keep in the fridge.

Tip: Save the chicken for a delicious salad or to add back into the stock to make a chunky chicken soup. The stock can be kept for 3 days in the fridge/3 months in freezer in an airtight Tupperware box or Kilner jar - just skim off the fat when ready to use.

Per serving: Calories: 65; Fat: 1g; Carbohydrates: 2g; Phosphorus: 84mg; Potassium: 137mg; Sodium: 33mg; Protein: 11g

ROSEMARY AND LEMON CHICKEN WITH EGGPLANT

SERVES 4 / PREP TIME: 10 MINUTES / COOK TIME: 40 MINUTES

A herby and delicious roast dinner.

---

6 OZ SKINLESS CHICKEN BREASTS

1/2 WHITE ONION, ROUGHLY CHOPPED

2 GARLIC CLOVES, CHOPPED

1 CUP CUBED EGGPLANT

2 TBSP ROSEMARY, FRESH OR DRIED

A PINCH OF BLACK PEPPER

1/4 CUP WATER

1 TBSP EXTRA VIRGIN OLIVE OIL

1 TBSP BALSAMIC VINEGAR

1/2 LEMON

1 TBSP FRESH BASIL

---

1. Preheat the oven to 375°F/190°C/Gas Mark 5.
2. Add the chicken, onion, garlic and eggplant to a lined baking tray and sprinkle over the rosemary and black pepper.
3. Pour over the water, olive oil and balsamic vinegar, so that the chicken and vegetables are sitting in a shallow bath.
4. Add 1/2 lemon to the baking tray for flavor.
5. Bake in the oven for 35-40 minutes or until the chicken is completely cooked through.
6. Serve the chicken and eggplant with a sprinkle of freshly torn basil and a little extra black pepper to serve.

Per serving: Calories: 121; Fat: 5g; Carbohydrates: 6g; Phosphorus: 108mg; Potassium: 231mg; Sodium: 210mg; Protein: 13g

PARSLEY AND TURKEY CABBAGE WRAPS

SERVES 4 / PREP TIME: 15 MINUTES / COOK TIME: 45 MINUTES

Bite into these meaty treats, all wrapped in nature's finest!

---

4 MEDIUM GREEN CABBAGE LEAVES	1 MEDIUM RED BELL PEPPER, FINELY DICED
7 OZ GROUND LEAN TURKEY	1 TBSP PARSLEY
1/2 ONION, FINELY DICED	1 TSP CRACKED BLACK PEPPER

---

1. Preheat the oven to 375°F/190°C/Gas Mark 5.
2. Carefully pull off the cabbage leaves from the cabbage, wash and leave intact.
3. Mix the rest of the ingredients in a bowl and divide into quarters.
4. Take a cabbage leaf and add a quarter of the mixture to the end of the leaf.
5. Roll from the stuffing end until you've wrapped the leaf around the stuffing.
6. Pierce through the centre with a toothpick so that the wraps stay together.
7. Repeat for the rest of the mixture.
8. Add the cabbage rolls to an oven dish and pour 1/2 cup water into the bottom, cover with a lid and bake for 45 minutes or until turkey is completely cooked through.
9. Remove from the oven and serve.

Per serving: Calories: 106; Fat: 6g; Carbohydrates: 4g; Phosphorus: 105g; Potassium: 206mg; Sodium: 32mg; Protein: 9g

TURKEY AND COUSCOUS STUFFED BELL PEPPERS

SERVES 4 / PREP TIME: 5 MINUTES / COOK TIME: 40 MINUTES

This is a filling and healthy treat!

1/2 CUP DRIED COUSCOUS

2 SMALL RED BELL PEPPERS

4 OZ LEAN GROUND TURKEY

1/2 RED ONION, FINELY DICED

1 CLOVE GARLIC, MINCED

1/2 TSP CAYENNE PEPPER

1 TBSP PARSLEY

1 TSP BLACK PEPPER

1/2 LIME

---

1. Preheat the oven to 350°f/170°c/Gas Mark 4.
2. In a heatproof bowl or dish, pour 1/2 cup boiling water over the couscous, cover and allow to steam for 3 minutes or according to package directions
3. Meanwhile, slice each pepper in half lengthways.
4. Remove the seeds from the middle of the bell peppers and layer onto a baking tray.
5. Combine the turkey mince with the onion, garlic, herbs and spices.
6. Stuff the peppers with the mixture.
7. Add to the oven for 30-40 minutes or until turkey is cooked through.
8. Serve with a side of couscous and a squeeze of fresh lime.

Per serving: Calories: 143; Fat: 8g; Carbohydrates: 20g; Phosphorus: 79mg; Potassium: 190mg; Sodium: 22mg; Protein: 8g

ZESTY CARIBBEAN CHICKEN

SERVES 4 / PREP TIME: 5 MINUTES / COOK TIME: 40 MINUTES

An exotic twist on your average chicken dish.

---

1 TBSP COCONUT OIL

1 TBSP HONEY

1 TBSP MUSTARD

2 TSP CURRY POWDER

1 GARLIC CLOVE, MINCED

1 TBSP JAMAICAN SPICE BLEND/ALL-SPICE

4X SMALL SKINLESS CHICKEN THIGHS

3/4 CUP WHITE RICE

1/2 CUP FRESH OR FROZEN GREEN PEAS

1 LIME

---

1. Preheat the oven to 350°f/170°c/Gas Mark 4.
2. Allow coconut oil to melt by warming in your hands or for a few seconds in a pan over the stove.
3. In a separate bowl, prepare marinade by mixing melted coconut oil, honey, mustard, garlic, and spices.
4. Pour over the chicken into a baking dish.
5. Place in the oven for 35-40 minutes.
6. Meanwhile, prepare your rice: bring a pan of water to the boil, add rice, cover and simmer for 20 minutes.
7. Add the peas to the pan in the last 5 minutes of cooking time.
8. Drain and cover the rice and return to the stove for 5 minutes.
9. When chicken is cooked through, serve on a bed of rice and peas and squeeze fresh lime juice over the top.
10. Enjoy.

Per serving: Calories: 220; Fat: 8g; Carbohydrates: 24g; Phosphorus: 172mg; Potassium: 293mg; Sodium: 210mg; Protein: 15g

CAJUN CHICKEN AND SHRIMP FIESTA

SERVES 4 / PREP TIME: 10 MINUTES / COOK TIME: 40 MINUTES

Absolutely delicious!

FOR THE CAJUN SPICE BLEND:

1 TSP CAYENNE PEPPER

1 TSP PAPRIKA

1 TSP DRIED OREGANO

1 TSP DRIED THYME

1 TBSP EXTRA VIRGIN OLIVE OIL

2 3OZ SKINLESS CHICKEN BREASTS, CHOPPED

1 WHITE ONION, CHOPPED

1 GARLIC CLOVE, CRUSHED

8 FRESH OR FROZEN LARGE SHRIMP

1 RED BELL PEPPER, CHOPPED

3/4 CUP WHITE RICE

1 CUP WATER

---

1. Mix the spices and herbs in a bowl to form your Cajun spice blend.
2. Grab a large pan and heat the olive oil on a medium to high heat.
3. Add the chicken and brown for around 4-5 minutes.
4. Remove chicken and place to one side.
5. Add the onion to the pan and fry until soft.
6. Now add the garlic, shrimp, Cajun seasoning and red pepper to the pan and cook for around 5 minutes or until prawns turn opaque.
7. Add the rice along with the chicken and water to the pan.
8. Cover the pan and simmer for around 25 minutes or until the rice is soft and the chicken is cooked through.
9. Serve hot!

Tip: multiply the quantities of the spices to make a Cajun spice mix that you can use again –just keep in a sealable jar or Tupperware somewhere dry!

Per serving: Calories: 186; Fat: 8g; Carbohydrates: 17g; Phosphorus: 160mg; Potassium: 315mg; Sodium: 310mg; Protein: 17g

HOMEMADE TURKEY BURGERS

SERVES 2 / PREP TIME: 15 MINUTES / COOK TIME: 35 MINUTES

Juicy turkey burgers for lunch or dinner.

1/2 WHITE ONION, FINELY DICED

1 CELERY STALK, FINELY DICED

1/2 RED BELL PEPPER, FINELY DICED

2 TBSP OLIVE OIL

PINCH OF BLACK PEPPER TO TASTE

1 TSP DILL

1 TSP CILANTRO

1 TSP DRY MUSTARD

3 OZ LEAN GROUND TURKEY MEAT

2 HAMBURGER ROLLS

1/2 CUP ARUGULA/BABY SPINACH

---

1. Pre-heat oven to 400°F/200 °C/Gas Mark 6.
2. Mix the vegetables, olive oil, pepper, herbs, and mustard in a medium bowl.
3. Add the meat to the vegetables and mix together until combined.
4. Use wet hands to 2 create burger patties.
5. Place the burgers on a lightly oiled baking tray and bake in the oven for 25-30 minutes or until meat is cooked through (use a knife in the center to check; the juices should run clear).
6. Serve in the hamburger roll and top with arugula/spinach and a helping of extra mustard as desired.

Per serving: Calories: 325; Fat: 20g; Carbohydrates: 23g; Phosphorus: 157mg; Potassium: 385mg; Sodium: 229mg; Protein: 15g

SPICY CHICKEN FAJITAS

SERVES 6 / PREP TIME: 5 MINUTES / COOK TIME: 15 MINUTES

Marvellously Mexican!

- 6 FLOUR 4" TORTILLAS
- 1/4 CUP GREEN PEPPER
- 1/4 CUP RED PEPPER
- 1/2 CUP ONION
- 2/3 CUP GREEN ONIONS, SLICED
- 2 TBSP CANOLA OIL
- 6 OZ BONELESS CHICKEN BREASTS

- 1/4 TSP BLACK PEPPER
- 1 TSP CHILI POWDER
- 1/2 TSP CUMIN
- 1/2 CUP CILANTRO
- 2 TBSP LEMON JUICE

---

1. Preheat oven to 300°F/150 °C/Gas Mark 2.
2. Wrap tortillas in foil and heat through in the oven for 10 minutes.
3. Meanwhile, chop the peppers, onions, and cilantro.
4. Cut chicken breasts into thin strips.
5. Place oil in a skillet over a medium heat.
6. Add the chicken, pepper, spices and lemon juice. Cook for 5-6 minutes.
7. Add the peppers and onion to the skillet and cook for a further 4 to 5 minutes or until chicken is completely cooked through.
8. Sprinkle the cilantro and squeeze the lemon juice over the chicken and fill the tortillas before wrapping.
9. Serve hot!

Per serving: Calories: 141; Fat: 7g; Carbohydrates: 10g; Phosphorus: 104mg; Potassium: 220mg; Sodium: 248mg; Protein: 10g

GINGER AND SCALLION CHICKEN STIR FRY

SERVES 4 / PREP TIME: 5 MINUTES / COOK TIME: 30 MINUTES

Fresh and aromatic!

---

2 CUP RICE NOODLES, UNSALTED

1 TBSP COCONUT OIL

2X 3OZ SKINLESS CHICKEN BREASTS

1 CARROT, PEELED AND CHOPPED

1/4 CUP CELERY, CHOPPED

1/2 CUP CHESTNUT MUSHROOMS

1/2 CUP SCALLIONS, CHOPPED

1 TBSP FRESH GINGER, GRATED

1 GARLIC CLOVE, MINCED

1 LIME

---

1. Boil a pan of water on a high heat and add noodles. Cook for 10-15 minutes or according to package guidelines.
2. Meanwhile, heat oil in a wok on a high heat and add chopped chicken breasts.
3. Sauté for 15-20 minutes or until thoroughly cooked and place to one side.
4. Now add the carrot, celery and chestnut mushrooms to the same wok and cook for 10 minutes before adding scallions, ginger, garlic and cooked chicken back into the pan.
5. Stir through for a few minutes until piping hot throughout and add noodles to the wok after draining.
6. Serve with the juice of your lime squeezed over the top.

Per serving: Calories: 323; Fat: 6g; Carbohydrates: 52g; Phosphorus: 158mg; Potassium: 309mg; Sodium: 263g; Protein: 15g

DEEP SOUTH CHICKEN STEW

SERVES 6 / PREP TIME: 10 MINUTES / COOK TIME: 40 MINUTES

Warms the soul!

3 CUPS COOKED WHITE RICE

2 TBSP CANOLA OIL

6 CHICKEN DRUMSTICKS

1/2 CUP ONION, SLICED

3/4 CUP GREEN BELL PEPPER, SLICED

2 TBSP ALL-PURPOSE FLOUR

3 GARLIC CLOVES, MINCED

1/4 TSP BLACK PEPPER

1 DASH RED PEPPER

1/2 CUP HOMEMADE CHICKEN STOCK

1/2 CUP WATER

1. Prepare rice according to package directions (without salt).
2. Heat oil in a large pot over a medium to high heat.
3. Add chicken pieces to the skillet and brown on each side.
4. Add the onion and green pepper to the pan.
5. Sprinkle the flour over the ingredients in the skillet and stir to coat for a further 5 minutes.
6. Now add the garlic, black pepper, and red pepper.
7. Stir in the stock and water.
8. Cover pot and allow to simmer for approximately 30 minutes or until chicken is fully cooked and stock has thickened.
9. Serve over white rice.

Per serving: Calories: 249; Fat: 8g; Carbohydrates: 27g; Phosphorus: 164mg; Potassium: 260mg; Sodium: 73 mg; Protein: 15g

HARISSA SPICED CHICKEN TRAY-BAKE

SERVES 4 / PREP TIME: 15 MINUTES / COOK TIME: 30 MINUTES

A week night staple in any home.

---

6 OZ SKINLESS CHICKEN BREASTS

1 SPAGHETTI SQUASH, CHOPPED AND PEELED

1 RED ONION, ROUGHLY CHOPPED

FOR THE HARISSA PASTE:

1 RED BELL PEPPER, DICED

1 TSP DRIED RED CHILLI

1 GARLIC CLOVE, MINCED
1 TSP CARAWAY SEEDS, CRUSHED

1 TSP GROUND CUMIN

1 TSP FRESH OR DRIED CILANTRO

2 TBSP EXTRA VIRGIN OLIVE OIL

---

1. Combine harissa spices and olive oil in a bowl.
2. Coat the chicken breast and vegetables with the harissa paste, cover and allow to marinate in the fridge for as long as possible.
3. When ready to cook, preheat oven to 375°F/190 °C/Gas Mark 5.
4. Add chicken to a baking tray and place in the oven to bake for 30 minutes.
5. Serve hot.

Top tip: Double up the Harissa spices and save some for cooking later on – it tastes great on fish, chicken, turkey and even simple roasted Mediterranean vegetables.

Per serving: Calories: 187; Fat: 9g; Carbohydrates: 13g; Phosphorus: 137mg; Potassium: 399mg; Sodium: 224mg; Protein: 14g

CHICKEN WITH SPICED RED CABBAGE AND CRANBERRY SAUCE

SERVES 4 / PREP TIME: 2 MINUTES / COOK TIME: 30 MINUTES

Hearty and delicious!

---

1 RED CABBAGE, SLICED AND SOAKED IN WARM WATER

1 TBSP NUTMEG

1 TBSP EXTRA VIRGIN OLIVE OIL

1/4 RED ONION, FINELY SLICED

6 OZ SKINLESS, CHICKEN BREASTS, SLICED

1 CUP CRANBERRIES

1 TBSP APPLE VINEGAR

1 TSP BROWN SUGAR

---

1. Bring a pan of water to boiling point and add the sliced red cabbage with the nutmeg to the water.
2. Cover and simmer for 15-20 minutes.
3. Meanwhile, heat the oil in a skillet on a medium to high heat.
4. Add the onions and sauté for 5-6 minutes until soft.
5. Now add the chicken breasts for 10 minutes on each side.
6. In a separate small pan, add the cranberries with water to cover and the apple vinegar and brown sugar.
7. Bring to a boil and then turn down heat and simmer for 10 minutes or until cranberries are soft. Keep an eye on water levels and top up if necessary.
8. Once the cranberries are soft, blend in a food processor until smooth.
9. Drain the cabbage and season with black pepper.
10. Serve chicken breast on a bed of red cabbage and drizzle cranberry sauce over to taste.

Per serving: Calories: 213; Fat: 6g; Carbohydrates: 28g; Phosphorus: 121mg; Potassium: 298mg; Sodium: 235 mg; Protein: 14g

AROMATIC CHICKEN AND EGGPLANT CURRY

SERVES 4 / PREP TIME: 10 MINUTES / COOK TIME: 35 MINUTES

Exotic flavors combine in this delightful curry.

---

1 TBSP COCONUT OIL

1/2 WHITE ONION, DICED

1 TSP GARAM MASALA

1 TSP CUMIN

1 TSP TURMERIC

1 CLOVE GARLIC, MINCED

1/2 CUP CHOPPED TOMATOES, NO ADDED SALT OR SUGAR

1 CUP WATER

2X 2 OZ SKINLESS CHICKEN BREASTS, CHOPPED

1 CUP EGGPLANT, SOAKED IN WARM WATER AND CUBED

2 CUPS WHITE RICE

2 TBSP FRESH CILANTRO, FINELY CHOPPED

---

1. Heat oil in a pan on a medium heat and add onions, stirring for 3-4 minutes until they begin to soften.
2. Add spices one by one and stir for 4-5 minutes, releasing the flavors.
3. Now add the garlic and stir.
4. Add the tomatoes and water to the pan and stir thoroughly.
5. Now add the chicken pieces and eggplant, cover and simmer for 25-30 minutes until chicken is completely cooked through.
6. Meanwhile prepare your rice by bringing a pan of water to the boil, before adding rice and covering to simmer for 20 minutes.
7. Drain and cover the rice and return to the stove for 5 minutes.
8. Serve individual rice portions and the chicken curry over the top.
9. Sprinkle with fresh cilantro to serve.

Per serving: Calories: 200; Fat: 5g; Carbohydrates: 27g; Phosphorus: 117mg; Potassium: 264mg; Sodium: 144mg; Protein: 11g

ITALIAN CHICKEN

SERVES 4 / PREP TIME: 10 MINUTES / COOK TIME: 20 MINUTES

A herby, tasty treat!

---

1 TSP DRIED THYME

1 TSP DRIED ROSEMARY

1 TSP DRIED BASIL

2X 3OZ SKINLESS CHICKEN BREASTS

1 TBSP OLIVE OIL

1 GARLIC CLOVE, MINCED

1/2 LEMON

1 TSP BLACK PEPPER

---

1. Combine herbs in a bowl.
2. Place 1 chicken breast onto a chopping board, sprinkle with 1/2 herb mix and cover with plastic wrap; use a meat pounder or rolling pin to flatten the chicken breast.
3. Repeat for the remaining chicken breasts and herb mix.
4. Heat half the oil in a non-stick pan over a medium heat and add chicken breasts.
5. Cook for 8 minutes on each side until thoroughly cooked through.
6. Add garlic to the pan and stir for 2 minutes.
7. In a dressing bowl, whisk lemon juice, the rest of the olive oil and black pepper.
8. Drizzle the lemon dressing over the chicken breasts to serve with your favorite rice or couscous and greens.

Per serving: Calories: 104; Fat: 5g; Carbohydrates: 2g; Phosphorus: 101mg; Potassium: 188mg; Sodium: 208 mg; Protein: 13g

ORANGE & GINGER CHICKEN NOODLES

SERVES 2 / PREP TIME: 5 MINUTES / COOK TIME: 20 MINUTES

Fresh and zesty noodles.

1 CUP RICE/BUCKWHEAT NOODLES

2 TSP COCONUT OIL

3 OZ SKINLESS CHICKEN BREAST, CHOPPED

1/2 CUP SCALLIONS, CHOPPED AND SOAKED IN WARM WATER

1/4 CUP BEAN SPROUTS, SOAKED IN WARM WATER

1 THUMB SIZED PIECE OF GINGER, MINCED

1/2 ORANGE, JUICED

1 RADISH, SOAKED IN WARM WATER SLICED TO SERVE

1. Cook the rice/noodles in a pan of boiling water for 10-12 minutes or according to package instructions.
2. Meanwhile, heat 1 tsp oil in a skillet over a medium heat.
3. Sauté the chopped chicken breast for 10-15 minutes or until thoroughly cooked through.
4. Add the scallions and bean sprouts for the last 5 minutes and sauté.
5. In a separate bowl, mix together the ginger, 1 tsp oil and orange juice.
6. Once chicken and noodles are cooked and drained, add all of the cooked ingredients along with the sliced radish to the dressing and toss through.
7. Serve warm or chilled.

Tip: Layer a mason jar or sealable container so you can enjoy your delicious, healthy lunch on the go.

Tip 2: Use lime instead of orange if you have been advised not to include oranges in your diet - check with your doctor if unsure.

Per serving: Calories: 344; Fat: 7g; Carbohydrates: 54g; Phosphorus: 157mg; Potassium: 345mg; Sodium: 250mg; Protein: 15g

LEBANESE·CHICKEN KEBABS AND RED ONION SALSA

SERVES 4 / PREP TIME: 15 MINUTES / COOK TIME: 25 MINUTES

Succulent spicy chicken with a cooling salsa.

FOR THE CHICKEN:

2 TBSP LEMON JUICE

4 GARLIC CLOVES, MINCED

1 TBSP THYME, FINELY CHOPPED

1 TBSP PAPRIKA

2 TSP GROUND CUMIN

1 TSP CAYENNE PEPPER

6OZ SKINLESS CHICKEN BREASTS, CUBED
4 METAL KEBAB SKEWERS

FOR THE SALSA:

1 RED ONION, FINELY DICED

1 RED BELL PEPPER, FINELY DICED

1 TBSP EXTRA VIRGIN OLIVE OIL

1 LIME, JUICED

1 TSP BLACK PEPPER

1 TBSP FRESH CILANTRO, FINELY CHOPPED

LEMON WEDGES TO GARNISH

1. Whisk the lemon juice, garlic, thyme, paprika, cumin, and cayenne pepper in a bowl.
2. Skewer the chicken cubes using kebab sticks (metal).
3. Baste the chicken on each side with the marinade, covering for as long as possible in the fridge (the lemon juice will tenderize the meat which is great for anti-inflammation, one of the symptoms of kidney disease).
4. When ready to cook, preheat the oven to 400°F/200 °C/Gas Mark 6 and bake for 20-25 minutes or until chicken is thoroughly cooked through.
5. Prepare the salsa by mixing all salsa ingredients in a separate bowl.
6. Serve the chicken kebabs, garnished with the lemon wedges and the salsa on the side.

Per serving: Calories: 148; Fat: 6g; Carbohydrates: 11g; Phosphorus: 139mg; Potassium: 396mg; Sodium: 213 mg; Protein: 14g

MEDITERRANEAN CHICKEN AND ZUCCHINI PASTA

SERVES 4 / PREP TIME: 1 HOUR / COOK TIME: 30 MINUTES

Zucchini pasta is so delicious and pairs excellently with the chicken.

FOR THE CHICKEN:

2X 2 OZ SKINLESS CHICKEN BREASTS, SLICED

2 TBSP EXTRA VIRGIN OLIVE OIL

JUICE OF 1/2 LEMON

1 CLOVE GARLIC, CRUSHED

1/2 TSP DRIED OREGANO

PINCH OF BLACK PEPPER

FOR THE PASTA:

3 ZUCCHINIS,

1 TSP EXTRA VIRGIN OLIVE OIL

---

1. Marinate the chicken slices in 1 tbsp. olive oil, lemon, garlic, oregano and pepper for at least 1 hour and up to overnight.
2. Pre-heat oven to 400°F/200°C/Gas Mark 6 when ready to cook.
3. Line a baking sheet with foil or parchment paper.
4. Layer the chicken strips on the baking tray and cook for 20-25 minutes or until cooked through.
5. Meanwhile, prepare your zucchini by slicing into thin spaghetti strips – use a mandolin or spiralizer and leave in a colander to drain for 10 minutes.
6. When chicken is cooked through, remove from oven and place to one side.
7. Boil a pan of water on a medium heat and add a pinch of black pepper.
8. Add your zucchini spaghetti to the water and boil for 2 minutes before immediately draining.
9. Plate and serve, layering the chicken on top and drizzling with 1 tsp. olive oil and a little black pepper.

Tip: If you're in a rush this will still taste delicious without the marinating time, just coat your chicken and cook straight away.

Per serving: Calories: 144; Fat: 9g; Carbohydrates: 6g; Phosphorus: 119mg; Potassium: 371mg; Sodium: 140mg; Protein: 10g

WALNUT AND BASIL CHICKEN DELIGHT

SERVES 2 / PREP TIME: 10 MINUTES / COOK TIME: 35 MINUTES

Making your own pesto tastes so much more delightful and means you can control the ingredients going in – ideal for those on a renal diet! Just keep an eye on your potassium and sodium intake because of the walnuts.

3OZ SKINLESS CHICKEN BREAST

1/4 CUP CRUSHED WALNUTS

1/2 CUP ARUGULA

1 BUNCH OF FRESH BASIL

1/2 CUP RAW SPINACH

2 TBSP EXTRA VIRGIN OLIVE OIL

1/4 CUP BRIE (OPTIONAL)

---

1. Preheat oven to 350°f/170°c/Gas Mark 4.
2. Take the chicken breasts and use a meat pounder to 'thin' each breast into 1cm thick escalopes.
3. Reserve a handful of the nuts and arugula.
4. Add the rest of the ingredients and a little black pepper to a blender or pestle and mortar and blend until smooth (you can leave this a little chunky for a rustic feel if you wish).
5. Add a little water if the pesto needs thinning.
6. Coat the chicken in the pesto.
7. Bake the chicken in the oven for at least 30 minutes or until chicken is completely cooked through.
8. Top each chicken escalope with the remaining nuts and place under the broiler for 5 minutes for a crispy topping to complete.
9. Serve on a bed of arugula.

Per serving: Calories: 321; Fat: 29g; Carbohydrates: 3g; Phosphorus: 159mg; Potassium: 257mg; Sodium: 137mg; Protein: 15g

CHINESE CHICKEN

SERVES 6 / PREP TIME: 5 MINUTES COOK TIME: 20 MINUTES

Quick and easy stir fry!

---

8 OZ LO MIEN NOODLES

2 TBSP OLIVE OIL

6 OZ BONELESS, SKINLESS, CHICKEN BREASTS, SLICED

1 CUP ONION, SLICED

1-1/2 CUPS CARROTS, SLICED

1 CUP CELERY, SLICED

1 CUP MUSHROOMS, SLICED

1 TBSP REDUCED-SODIUM SOY SAUCE

---

1. Bring a pan of water to the boil and cook noodles for 10-12 minutes or according to package directions.
2. Drain and place to one side.
3. Heat olive oil in a wok or skillet over a medium to high heat.
4. Add chicken and sauté for 10-15 minutes.
5. Ensure chicken has turned white on each side.
6. Now add onions, carrots, and celery.
7. Stir-fry gently for 5 minutes.
8. Add the mushrooms, soy sauce and drained noodles, stirring until heated through.
9. Ensure chicken is completely cooked through.

Per serving: Calories: 187; Fat: 6g; Carbohydrates: 22g; Phosphorus: 155mg; Potassium: 392mg; Sodium: 283 mg; Protein: 13g

MEATS
(BEEF, PORK & LAMB)

HOMEMADE BURGERS

SERVES 2 / PREP TIME: 10 MINUTES / COOK TIME: 20 MINUTES

Succulent beef burgers, oozing with brie cheese and mustard.

---

4 OZ LEAN 100% GROUND BEEF

1 TSP BLACK PEPPER

1 GARLIC CLOVE, MINCED

1 TSP OLIVE OIL

1/4 CUP ONION, FINELY DICED

1 TBSP BALSAMIC VINEGAR

1/2OZ BRIE CHEESE, CRUMBLED

1 TSP MUSTARD

---

1. Season ground beef with pepper and then mix in minced garlic.
2. Form burger shapes with the ground beef using the palms of your hands.
3. Heat a skillet on a medium to high heat, and then add the oil.
4. Sauté the onions for 5-10 minutes until browned.
5. Then add the balsamic vinegar and sauté for another 5 minutes.
6. Remove and set aside.
7. Add the burgers to the pan and heat on the same heat for 5-6 minutes before flipping and heating for a further 5-6 minutes until cooked through.
8. Spread the mustard onto each burger.
9. Crumble the brie cheese over each burger and serve!
10. Try with a crunchy side salad!

Tip: If using fresh beef and not defrosted, prepare double the ingredients and freeze burgers in plastic wrap (after cooling) for up to 1 month.
Thoroughly defrost before heating through completely in the oven to serve.

Per serving: Calories: 178; Fat: 10g; Carbohydrates: 4g; Phosphorus: 147mg; Potassium: 272mg; Sodium: 273 mg; Protein: 16g

SLOW-COOKED BEEF BRISKET

SERVES 6 / PREP TIME: 10 MINUTES / COOK TIME: 3.5 HOURS

Melt in the mouth beef stew, so easily prepared!

10 OZ CHUCK ROAST	2 GARLIC CLOVES
1 ONION, SLICED	2 TBSP EXTRA VIRGIN OLIVE OIL
1 CUP CARROTS, PEELED AND SLICED	1 TSP BLACK PEPPER
1 TBSP MUSTARD	1 CUP HOMEMADE CHICKEN STOCK (p.52)
1 TBSP THYME (FRESH OR DRIED)	1 CUP WATER
1 TBSP ROSEMARY (FRESH OR DRIED)	

1. Preheat oven to 300°f/150°c/Gas Mark 2.
2. Trim any fat from the beef and soak vegetables in warm water.
3. Make a paste by mixing together the mustard, thyme, rosemary, and garlic, before mixing in the oil and pepper.
4. Combine this mix with the stock.
5. Pour the mixture over the beef into an oven proof baking dish.
6. Place the vegetables onto the bottom of the baking dish with the beef.
7. Cover and roast for 3 hours, or until tender.
8. Uncover the dish and continue to cook for 30 minutes in the oven.
9. Serve hot!

Tip: Prepare this meal in a slow cooker overnight instead! Just follow instructions 1-6 and then pour into the slow cooker dish and set to low.

Per serving: Calories: 151; Fat: 7g; Carbohydrates: 7g; Phosphorus: 144mg; Potassium: 344mg ; Sodium: 279mg; Protein: 15g

APRICOT AND LAMB TAGINE

SERVES 3 / PREP TIME: 10 MINUTES / COOK TIME:1-1.5 HOURS

Aromatic and wonderful!

---

1 TBSP OF EXTRA VIRGIN OLIVE OIL

2 LEAN LAMB FILLETS, CUBED

1/2 ONION, DICED

1 TSP CUMIN

1 TSP TURMERIC

1 TSP CURRY POWDER

1 CUP OF HOMEMADE CHICKEN STOCK (p.52) OR WATER

1 TSP DRIED ROSEMARY

1/2 CUP CANNED APRICOTS, JUICES DRAINED AND APRICOTS RINSED

1 TSP OF CHOPPED PARSLEY

---

1. Heat the olive oil in a large oven-proof pot over a medium high heat on the stove.
2. Add the lamb to the pot and cook for 5 minutes until browned.
3. Remove lamb and place to one side.
4. Add the chopped onion to the pot and sauté for 5 minutes until starting to soften.
5. Sprinkle the cumin, turmeric and curry powder over the onions and continue to stir for 4-5 minutes.
6. Now add the lamb back into the pot with the chicken stock and rosemary.
7. Then cover the pot and leave to simmer on a low heat for 1-1.5 hours until the lamb is tender and fully cooked through.
8. Add the apricots 15 minutes before the end of the cooking time.
9. Plate up and serve with the chopped parsley to garnish.

Tip: Follow instructions 1-5 and then complete the remaining steps in a slow cooker/Dutch oven and leave on a medium heat overnight.

Per serving: Calories: 194; Fat: 9g; Carbohydrates: 13g; Phosphorus: 140mg; Potassium: 372mg ; Sodium: 197mg; Protein: 15g

LEMONGRASS AND COCONUT BEEF CURRY

SERVES 5 / PREP TIME: 10 MINUTES / COOK TIME: 45 MINUTES

Fresh, zingy and hot all at the same time!

1 TBSP COCONUT OIL

2 GARLIC CLOVES, MINCED

6 OZ 100% GRASS-FED SIRLOIN, SLICED INTO STRIPS AND FAT TRIMMED

1 TSP OF FRESH GINGER, GRATED

1 TSP CURRY POWDER

1 STICK OF LEMONGRASS, VERY FINELY DICED

1/4 CUP OF HOMEMADE CHICKEN STOCK (p.52)

1 CUP OF TENDER-STEM OR SPROUTING BROCCOLI

1/2 WHITE ONION, CHOPPED

1/2 CUP LOW FAT COCONUT MILK

1 STEM OF GREEN ONION, SLICED

1 1/2 CUPS COOKED BROWN RICE/WHITE RICE (CHECK WHAT YOUR DIETITIAN RECOMMENDS)

1. Heat the coconut oil and garlic in a large pan over a medium to high heat for 2 minutes.
2. Add the beef slices to the pan and brown each side for 2 minutes.
3. Once browned, remove beef from the pan and place to one side.
4. Mix the ginger, curry powder, lemongrass and ¼ of the homemade chicken stock in a separate bowl.
5. Pour the stock mix, along with the broccoli into the pan.
6. Add the beef back into the pan along with the chopped onions.
7. Add the last of the stock and coconut milk over the beef and simmer for 30-40 minutes or until piping hot and the beef is soft.
8. Serve piping hot with the green onion scattered over the top and rice on the side.

Tip: Check with your doctor or dietitian as to whether you can still have coconut milk. Alternatively use a non-dairy milk such as almond.

Per serving: Calories: 239; Fat: 11g; Carbohydrates: 26g; Phosphorus: 179mg; Potassium: 364mg ; Sodium: 42mg; Protein: 11g

CHILI CRISPY BEEF NOODLES

SERVES 4 / PREP TIME: 10 MINUTES / COOK TIME: 10-12 HOURS IN SLOW COOKER

Sticky, crispy and delicious!

FOR THE BEEF:

1/2 SMALL WHITE ONION

1 GARLIC CLOVE, MINCED

2 TBSP FRESH PARSLEY

8 OZ CHUCK ROAST, BONELESS & FAT TRIMMED

5 CUPS WATER

1 BAY LEAF

1 TSP BLACK PEPPER

8 OZ RICE NOODLES

FOR THE CHILI SEASONING:

2 TBSP OLIVE OIL

1 TBSP CHILI FLAKES

1 GARLIC CLOVE, MINCED

TO SERVE:

1 STEM GREEN ONION, FINELY CHOPPED

1 LIME

---

1. Add all of the ingredients for the beef (up to and including black pepper) to a crock pot or slow cooker and cook on a medium heat for 10-12 hours or until very tender.
2. Remove the beef and shred the meat with a fork.
3. Cook noodles in a pot of boiling water for 10-15 minutes or according to package directions.
4. Whisk the olive oil, chili flakes, and garlic and add to a pan on a high heat.
5. Add the beef to the hot chili seasoning and cook on a high heat for 8-10 minutes or until crispy.
6. Scatter the green onions over the beef and stir.
7. Remove from the pan and portion over the noodles.
8. Squeeze the lime juice over the top to serve.

Per serving: Calories: 415; Fat: 17g; Carbohydrates: 51g; Phosphorus: 125mg; Potassium: 194mg ; Sodium: 138mg; Protein: 14g

HARISSA LAMB BURGERS WITH YOGURT AND CUMIN DIP

SERVES 2 / PREP TIME: 10 MINUTES / COOK TIME: 20 MINUTES

Moroccan spiced lamb burgers.

---

5 OZ LEAN GROUND LAMB

1/4 CUP RED ONION, FINELY DICED

1 TBSP PARSLEY

1 TSP HARISSA SPICES

1 CLOVE OF GARLIC, MINCED

1 TBSP EXTRA VIRGIN OLIVE OIL

1/2 CUP ARUGULA

1/4 LEMON, JUICED

1 TSP CUMIN

1/2 CUP NON-DAIRY YOGURT SUCH AS ALMOND TO SERVE (OPTIONAL)

---

1. Preheat the broiler on a medium to high heat.
2. Mix together the ground lamb, red onion, parsley, Harissa spices, garlic and olive oil until combined.
3. Shape 1 inch thick patties using wet hands.
4. Add the patties to a baking tray and place under the broiler for 7-8 minutes on each side or until thoroughly cooked through.
5. Plate up each burger and top with a helping of arugula.
6. Whisk the lemon juice and cumin and drizzle over the arugula topped burgers.

Tip: Mix a non-dairy yogurt such as almond yogurt with the cumin and lemon juice for a refreshing dip!

Per serving: Calories: 208; Fat: 16g; Carbohydrates: 4g; Phosphorus: 110mg; Potassium: 255mg ; Sodium: 43mg; Protein: 12g

MIGHTY MEATLOAF

SERVES 4 / PREP TIME: 10 MINUTES / COOK TIME: 30 MINUTES

Delicious!

1/2 WHITE ONION, DICED

2 GARLIC CLOVES, MINCED

1 ZUCCHINI, GRATED

2 TBSP EXTRA VIRGIN OLIVE OIL

1 TBSP CHOPPED FRESH OR DRIED PARSLEY

7 OZ GROUND LEAN PORK

1/2 CUP JARRED RED BELL PEPPERS, CHOPPED

1/4 CUP LOW FAT COCONUT MILK

2 LARGE EGG WHITES

1 TBSP ALL PURPOSE FLOUR

1 TSP GROUND BLACK PEPPER

---

1. Preheat oven to 400°f/200°c/Gas Mark 6.
2. Soak vegetables in warm water for 10 minutes before draining.
3. Grease an oven-proof rectangular dish with 1 tbsp. olive oil.
4. Grab a skillet and heat 1 tbsp. oil on a medium heat.
5. Sauté the onion, garlic, zucchini with the parsley for five minutes, or until soft.
6. Place to one side to cool.
7. Add the pork, chopped peppers, coconut milk, egg whites, flour and black pepper to the vegetables and mix to combine.
8. Add the mixture to the oven dish and flatten the surface with a spoon.
9. Bake in the oven for 30 minutes or until thoroughly cooked through.
10. Remove and slice before serving with your choice of side dish.

Tip: Check with your doctor or dietitian as to whether you can still have coconut milk. Alternatively use a non-dairy milk such as almond.

Per serving: Calories: 248; Fat: 18g; Carbohydrates: 7g; Phosphorus: 145mg; Potassium: 403mg ; Sodium: 258mg; Protein: 16g

PULLED PORK AND APPLE BUNS

SERVES 4 / PREP TIME: 15 MINUTES / COOK TIME: 3-4 HOURS

Sweet and Savory.

1/2 ONION, SLICED

3 CLOVES GARLIC

8 OZ BONELESS PORK SHOULDER ROAST

1 TBSP EXTRA VIRGIN OLIVE OIL

1 CUP WATER

1 TBSP RED WINE VINEGAR

1 TSP BLACK PEPPER

2 COOKING APPLES, PEELED AND

CHOPPED

3 TBSP BROWN SUGAR

4 BUNS TO SERVE

---

1. Preheat oven to 350°f/180°c/Gas Mark 5.
2. Soak the onion and garlic in warm water.
3. Meanwhile, cut the pork into cubes.
4. In a skillet, cook the pork, onions, and garlic in the oil over a medium heat for 5 minutes.
5. Into a baking dish, add the water, red wine vinegar, and black pepper.
6. Cover and bake for 3-4 hours.
7. Remove the cover and continue to cook for 30 minutes.
8. Meanwhile, add the apples and brown sugar to a pot over a high heat and cover with water, allowing to simmer for 15-20 minutes or until apples are soft.
9. Remove pork from the oven and allow to cool before shredding the meat with a fork.
10. Whiz up the apples in a blender and serve in the buns with the pulled pork.
11. Enjoy!

Per serving: Calories: 270; Fat: 12g; Carbohydrates: 29g; Phosphorus: 124mg; Potassium: 277mg ; Sodium: 168mg; Protein: 11g

MUSTARD AND LEEK PORK TENDERLOIN

SERVES 2 / PREP TIME: 10 MINUTES / COOK TIME: 35 MINUTES

Delicious!

---

1 TSP MUSTARD SEEDS	6 OZ PORK TENDERLOIN
1 TSP CUMIN SEEDS	1 TSP EXTRA VIRGIN OLIVE OIL
1 TSP DRY MUSTARD	1 LEEK, SLICED

---

1. Preheat the broiler to a medium to high heat.
2. In a dry skillet heat mustard and cumin seeds until they start to pop (3-5 minutes).
3. Grind seeds using a pestle and mortar or blender and then mix in the dry mustard.
4. Coat the pork on both sides with the mustard blend and add to a baking tray to broil for 25-30 minutes or until cooked through. Turn once halfway through.
5. Remove and place to one side.
6. Heat the oil in a pan on a medium heat and add the leeks for 5-6 minutes or until soft.
7. Slice and serve the pork tenderloin on a bed of leeks and enjoy!

Per serving: Calories: 165; Fat: 9g; Carbohydrates: 7g; Phosphorus: 154mg; Potassium: 309mg ; Sodium: 67mg; Protein: 14g

MALAYSIAN STYLE LAMB CURRY

SERVES 4 / PREP TIME: 10 MINUTES / COOK TIME: 1 HOUR

Scrumptious lamb dish.

---

1 TSP OLIVE OIL

1 ONION, DICED

6 OZ LEAN LAMB STEAKS, CUBED

1 CUP ALMOND OR RICE MILK (UNEN-RICHED)

1 TSP CURRY POWDER

1 EGGPLANT, ROUGHLY CHOPPED

1 TBSP CILANTRO

---

1. Heat oil in a pot over a medium to high heat and sauté onions for 5 minutes or until soft.
2. Add the lamb for 5-10 minutes, turning to brown each side, before adding the milk and curry powder.
3. Bring to the boil, then turn down the heat and add the eggplant to the curry.
4. Cover and simmer for 45-50 minutes or until the lamb is soft.
5. Scatter with cilantro and serve with rice or bread of your choice.

Tip: You could transfer the curry to a slow cooker and leave overnight to free you up from the stove if you wish - just ensure the liquid fully covers the lamb.

Tip: Double up on the ingredients and freeze in individual portions for an easy meal when you're too busy to cook!

Per serving: Calories: 166; Fat: 6g; Carbohydrates: 12g; Phosphorus: 133mg; Potassium: 329mg ; Sodium: 230mg; Protein: 15g

PORK CHOPS WITH RED CABBAGE AND CRANBERRY SAUCE

SERVES 4 / PREP TIME: 10 MINUTES / COOK TIME: 35 MINUTES

Delicious!

---

2 TSP CORNSTARCH

2 TSP HONEY

6OZ BONELESS PORK LOIN CHOPS, SLICED

1 TSP GROUND BLACK PEPPER

3/4 CUP CRANBERRIES

1/2 CUP WATER

1 CUP RED CABBAGE, SLICED

1 TSP CINNAMON

1 ORANGE

---

1. In a bowl, mix the cornstarch and honey until smooth.
2. Season the pork chops with the pepper.
3. Heat a skillet over a medium heat.
4. Sauté the pork slices until browned and cooked through (approximately 10 minutes or according to package directions).
5. Remove and place to one side.
6. Add the honey to the skillet and then the cranberries and water.
7. Bring to the boil, turn down the heat, and simmer for 10 minutes.
8. Meanwhile, bring a large pot of water to the boil, add the cabbage, cinnamon and orange juice.
9. Reduce heat and simmer for 10 minutes before draining.
10. Return the pork to the pan with the cranberries, cover and simmer for 5 minutes or until meat is piping hot throughout.
11. Serve pork on a bed of red cabbage and season with black pepper to taste.

Tip: Use lime instead of orange if you have been advised not to include oranges in your diet - check with your doctor if unsure.

Per serving: Calories: 142; Fat: 4g; Carbohydrates: 19g; Phosphorus: 126mg; Potassium: 365mg ; Sodium: 174mg; Protein: 13g

PARSLEY AND GARLIC MEATBALL SPAGHETTI

SERVES 3 / PREP TIME: 10 MINUTES / COOK TIME: 30 MINUTES

Lean pork meatballs, delicately flavored with Italian herbs.

3 OZ LEAN PORK MINCE

2 GARLIC CLOVES, CRUSHED

1/4 CUP 100% WHITE BREADCRUMBS

1 TBSP PARSLEY

FOR THE SAUCE:

1/2 TBSP EXTRA VIRGIN OLIVE OIL

1/2 CAN CHOPPED TOMATOES (NO ADDED SALT OR SUGAR)

1/2 CUP OF WATER

1/2 TBSP EXTRA VIRGIN OLIVE OIL

1/2 RED ONION, FINELY CHOPPED

1 CUP SPAGHETTI

1. Mix the pork mince with garlic, breadcrumbs and parsley in a bowl.
2. Season with a little black pepper and separate into 8 balls using your hands.
3. Heat 1/2 tbsp. oil in a pan over a medium heat and add onion, sautéing for a few minutes until softened.
4. Add the tomatoes and ½ cup water.
5. Cover and lower heat to simmer for 15 minutes.
6. Meanwhile, boil your water and cook spaghetti to recommended guidelines.
7. In a separate pan, heat 1/2 tbsp. oil and add the meatballs, turning carefully to brown the surface of each.
8. Continue this for 5-7 minutes before adding the meatballs to the sauce and simmering for a further 10 minutes.
9. Drain spaghetti, portion up and pour a half the meatballs and sauce over the top to serve.

Tip: If you are avoiding or limiting tomatoes, use a homemade vegetable or chicken stock instead.

Per serving: Calories: 333; Fat: 16g; Carbohydrates: 34g; Phosphorus: 146mg; Potassium: 355mg ; Sodium: 191mg; Protein: 13g

BEEF RAGU PASTA

SERVES 4 / PREP TIME: 15 MINUTES / COOK TIME: 1.5 HOURS

A rich Italian inspired pasta dish.

---

2 TBSP EXTRA VIRGIN OLIVE OIL

1/2 ONION, DICED

3 OZ TOPSIDE OF BEEF, CUBED

1/4 CAN CHOPPED TOMATOES (NO ADDED SALT OR SUGAR)

1 TBSP FRESH BASIL

1 CUP WATER

2 CUPS COOKED WHITE PASTA

1 TSP BLACK PEPPER

---

1. Over a medium heat, add oil to a pot and sauté the onion for 5 minutes or until soft.
2. Add the beef to the pan and brown each side.
3. Turn up the heat and add tomatoes, basil, and water, bring to a boil.
4. Turn down the heat, cover and simmer for 1.5 hours.
5. Serve over cooked pasta and season with black pepper.

Tip: If you are avoiding or limiting tomatoes, use a homemade vegetable or chicken stock instead.

Per serving: Calories: 306; Fat: 9g; Carbohydrates: 44; Phosphorus: 112mg; Potassium: 168mg ; Sodium: 29mg; Protein: 12g

ORIENTAL BEEF AND SPRING ONION WRAP

SERVES 2 / PREP TIME: 10 MINUTES / COOK TIME: 30 MINUTES

These delicious wraps are great for lunch or dinner and are loved by the whole family!

3 OZ LEAN GROUND BEEF	1 TSP GROUND GINGER
1 GARLIC CLOVE, MINCED	1 TSP CANOLA OIL
1 TBSP RICE WINE VINEGAR	1/2 CUCUMBER, DICED
1 TBSP CHILI FLAKES	2 ICEBERG LETTUCE LEAVES

1. Mix the ground meat with the garlic, rice wine vinegar, chili flakes and ginger in a bowl.
2. Heat oil in a skillet over a medium heat.
3. Add the beef to the pan and cook for 20-25 minutes or until cooked through.
4. Serve beef mixture with diced cucumber in each lettuce wrap and fold.

Per serving: Calories: 107; Fat: 5g; Carbohydrates: 4g; Phosphorus: 113mg; Potassium: 277mg; Sodium: 170mg; Protein: 12g

EGGPLANT MOUSSAKA

SERVES 4 / PREP TIME: 10 MINUTES / COOK TIME: 50 MINUTES

A Greek-inspired recipe.

1/2 WHITE ONION, DICED

1 GARLIC CLOVE, MINCED

8 OZ LEAN GROUND BEEF

1 TSP PARSLEY

1 TSP BLACK PEPPER

1 TSP CAYENNE PEPPER

1/2 CUP WATER

1 EGGPLANT, SLICED

FOR THE WHITE SAUCE:

1 TBSP UNSALTED BUTTER

2 TBSP ALL PURPOSE WHITE FLOUR

3/4 CUP RICE/ALMOND MILK (UNEN-RICHED)

1/4 TEASPOON WHITE PEPPER

1 TSP BLACK PEPPER

1. Preheat the oven to 350°f/170°c/Gas Mark 4.
2. Soak vegetables in warm water.
3. To prepare white sauce: Heat saucepan on a medium heat.
4. Add the butter to the pan on the side nearest to the handle.
5. Tilt the pan towards you and allow butter to melt.
6. Now add the flour to the opposite side of the pan and gradually mix the flour into the butter - continue to mix until smooth.
7. Add the milk and mix thoroughly for 10 minutes until lumps dissolve.
8. Add black pepper.
9. Turn off the heat and place to one side.
10. To prepare the moussaka: Spray a skillet with olive oil cooking spray on a medium to high heat and add onions and garlic for 5 minutes until soft.
11. Add lean beef mince, season with herbs and spices, add water and cook for 10-15 minutes or until completely browned.
12. Layer an ovenproof lasagna dish with 1/3 eggplant slices.
13. Add 1/3 beef mince on top.
14. Layer with 1/3 white sauce.
15. Repeat until ingredients are used.
16. Cover and add to the oven for 25-30 minutes or until golden and bubbly.
17. Remove and serve piping hot!

Per serving: Calories: 201; Fat: 13g; Carbohydrates: 7g; Phosphorus: 131mg; Potassium: 278mg ; Sodium: 267mg; Protein: 14g

BEEF RIBS AND HONEY

SERVES 2 / PREP TIME: 10 MINUTES / COOK TIME: 4 HOURS

A special treat.

4 OZ BEEF RIBS, TRIM TO 1/8"FAT	1 TSP BLACK PEPPER
1 TSP DRIED THYME	2 TBSP HONEY
1 TSP DRIED OREGANO	3 CUPS WATER
1 TSP DRIED PARSLEY	1 TBSP CIDER VINEGAR

1. Preheat the oven to 350°f/170°c/Gas Mark 4.
2. Sprinkle the ribs with the herbs and pepper.
3. Add the honey to coat.
4. Add water and vinegar to a baking dish and add the ribs.
5. Cover with aluminum foil and cook for 3-4 hours or until very tender.
6. Remove foil and continue cooking for 10 minutes.
7. Serve hot!

Per serving: Calories: 165; Fat:64g; Carbohydrates: 19g; Phosphorus: 81mg; Potassium: 148mg ; Sodium: 36mg; Protein: 10g

PEPPERED CREAMY BEEF AND RICE

SERVES 2 / PREP TIME: 10 MINUTES / COOK TIME: 4-5 HOURS

Healthy and filling.

---

1 TSP BLACK PEPPER

1 TSP DRIED OREGANO

1 GARLIC CLOVE, MINCED

1/2 ONION, DICED

1/2 CUP HOMEMADE CHICKEN STOCK (p.52)

2 OZ LEAN FRYING BEEF

2 TBSP WATER

2 TBSP ALL-PURPOSE WHITE FLOUR

2 TBSP LOW FAT SOUR CREAM

1 CUP WHITE/BROWN RICE (CHECK WHAT YOUR DIETITIAN RECOMMENDS)

---

1. Soak vegetables in warm water prior to cooking.
2. Into a slow cooker, add the pepper, oregano, garlic, onion, stock, and beef.
3. Cover and cook on high for 4-5 hours or until beef is tender.
4. Add the water, flour and sour cream to the crockpot and mix until smooth.
5. Continue to cook for another 20 minutes or until the mixture has thickened.
6. Meanwhile, bring a pan of water to the boil and add the rice for 20 minutes.
7. Drain the water from the rice, add the lid and steam for 5 minutes.
8. Serve the rice with the creamy beef over the top and enjoy!

Per serving: Calories: 240; Fat: 5g; Carbohydrates: 37g; Phosphorus: 199mg; Potassium: 334mg ; Sodium: 155mg; Protein: 14g

BEEF CHILI

SERVES 2 / PREP TIME: 10 MINUTES / COOK TIME: 30 MINUTES

A homemade favourite.

1/4 ONION, DICED

1 RED BELL PEPPER, DICED

2 GARLIC CLOVES, MINCED

1 CUP WHITE/BROWN RICE (CHECK WHAT YOUR DIETITIAN RECOMMENDS)

2 TBSP EXTRA VIRGIN OLIVE OIL

3 OZ LEAN GROUND BEEF

1 TSP CHILI POWDER

1 TSP OREGANO

1 CUP WATER

1 TBSP FRESH CILANTRO TO SERVE

---

1. Soak vegetables in warm water prior to cooking.
2. Bring a pan of water to the boil and add rice for 20 minutes.
3. Meanwhile, add the oil to a pan and heat on a medium to high heat.
4. Add the onions, pepper, and garlic and sauté for 5 minutes until soft.
5. Remove and set aside.
6. Add the beef to the pan and stir until browned.
7. Add the vegetables back into the pan and stir.
8. Now add the chili powder and herbs and the water, cover and turn the heat down a little to simmer for 15 minutes.
9. Meanwhile, drain the water from the rice, add the lid and steam while the chili is cooking.
10. Serve hot with the fresh cilantro sprinkled over the top.

Per serving: Calories: 326; Fat: 17g; Carbohydrates: 29g; Phosphorus: 198mg; Potassium: 343mg ; Sodium: 233mg; Protein: 14g

LAMB SHOULDER WITH ZUCCHINI AND EGGPLANT

SERVES 4 / PREP TIME: 10 MINUTES / COOK TIME: 4-5 HOURS

Sumptuous roasted lamb!

2 ZUCCHINIS, CUBED	1 TSP BLACK PEPPER
1 EGGPLANT, CUBED	1 TBSP BASIL
6 OZ LEAN LAMB SHOULDER	1 TBSP OREGANO
2 TBSP EXTRA VIRGIN OLIVE OIL	2 GARLIC CLOVES, CHOPPED

1. Preheat oven to its highest setting.
2. Soak the vegetables in warm water.
3. Trim any fat from the lamb shoulder.
4. Rub the lamb with 1 tbsp. olive oil, pepper and herbs.
5. Line a baking tray with the rest of the olive oil, garlic, zucchini and eggplant.
6. Add the lamb shoulder and cover with foil.
7. Turn the oven down to 325°f/170°c/Gas Mark 3 and add the dish into the oven.
8. Cook for 4-5 hours, remove and rest.
9. Slice the lamb with a carving knife and serve on a bed of the juicy roasted vegetables.

Per serving: Calories: 184; Fat: 12g; Carbohydrates: 9g; Phosphorus: 132mg; Potassium: 379mg ; Sodium: 101mg; Protein: 12g

SEAFOOD

SIZZLING SEA BASS

SERVES 2 / PREP TIME: 5 MINUTES / COOK TIME: 15 MINUTES

Hot, spicy and ready in a flash!

---

2 GREEN ONION STEMS, FINELY SLICED

1 TBSP EXTRA VIRGIN OLIVE OIL

1 TSP BLACK PEPPER

4 OZ SEA BASS FILLET

1 RED CHILI, DESEEDED AND THINLY SLICED

1 GARLIC CLOVE, THINLY SLICED

1 TSP GINGER, PEELED AND CHOPPED

---

1. Soak your green onions in warm water.
2. Meanwhile, grab a skillet and heat the oil over a medium to high heat.
3. Sprinkle black pepper over the sea bass fillet and score the skin of the fish a few times with a sharp knife.
4. Add the sea bass to the very hot pan with the skin side down.
5. Cook for 7-8 minutes and turn over (this will allow the skin to turn crispy and golden).
6. Cook for a further 3-4 minutes or until cooked through.
7. Remove sea bass from the skillet and allow to rest.
8. Add the chili, garlic, and ginger to the skillet and stir for approximately 2 minutes or until golden.
9. Remove from the heat and add the green onions.
10. Divide the sea bass into two portions.
11. Pour the vegetables over each portion of sea bass to serve.
12. Try with a side salad or rice.

Per serving: Calories: 116; Fat: 7g; Carbohydrates: 3g; Phosphorus: 70mg; Potassium: 179mg ; Sodium: 37mg; Protein: 10g

COOKED TILAPIA WITH MANGO SALSA

SERVES 2 / PREP TIME: 2 HOURS / COOK TIME: 10 MINUTES

A ceviche style dish which is easy to prepare and tastes great alone or with your favorite vegetables.

---

4 OZ FRESH TILAPIA FILLETS

1 LIME

1/2 RED BELL PEPPER, FINELY DICED

1/2 RED ONION, FINELY DICED

1 TBSP FRESH CILANTRO

1 TSP BLACK PEPPER

1/4 CUP OLIVE OIL

4 CRACKERS/SLICES OF MELBA TOAST

---

1. Preheat the broiler on a medium to high heat.
2. Cut tilapia into small bite size pieces.
3. Place tilapia under the broiler for 7-10 minutes or until cooked through.
4. Remove and allow to cool in a separate bowl, before squeezing the juice from the lime over the top and mixing well.
5. Mix the bell pepper, onion, cilantro, pepper and oil with the cooked tilapia and marinate for a minimum of 2 hours in the refrigerator.
6. Divide into two and serve with crackers/toast for a tasty lunch or starter.

Per serving: Calories: 376; Fat: 29g; Carbohydrates: 20g; Phosphorus: 135mg; Potassium: 370mg ; Sodium: 87mg; Protein: 13g

CILANTRO AND
CHILI INFUSED SWORDFISH

SERVES 2 / PREP TIME: 30 MINUTES / COOK TIME: 15 MINUTES

The meaty flavors combine deliciously with the fresh herbs and hot kick of the chili in this fish dish.

1/2 ONION, FINELY DICED	1 RED CHILI, FINELY DICED
4 OZ SWORDFISH FILLET	1 LEMON
2 TSP FRESH CILANTRO	1 TBSP EXTRA VIRGIN OLIVE OIL
1 TSP BROWN SUGAR	1 GARLIC CLOVE, MINCED

1. Soak the onion in warm water.
2. Meanwhile, add fish to an ovenproof baking dish.
3. Whisk cilantro, onion, sugar, chili, lemon juice, oil and garlic in a separate bowl.
4. Pour the marinade over the swordfish and turn to coat both sides.
5. Cover and marinate in the refrigerator at least 30 minutes.
6. Preheat the broiler to a medium heat when ready to cook.
7. Place oven dish under the broiler for 6-7 minutes on each side or until fish flakes easily with a fork.
8. Divide into two portions and serve with your choice of crisp green salad or vegetables.

Per serving: Calories: 171; Fat: 10g; Carbohydrates: 10g; Phosphorus: 152mg; Potassium: 349mg; Sodium: 43mg; Protein: 11g

CITRUS TUNA CEVICHE

SERVES 2 / PREP TIME: 2 MINUTES / COOK TIME: NA

Simple yet tasty!

---

4 OZ CAN LOW-SODIUM WATER-PACKED TUNA

1 TBSP CILANTRO

1 TSP BLACK PEPPER

1 LEMON

1 TSP RED WINE VINEGAR

1 RED BELL PEPPER, FINELY CHOPPED

1/2 RED ONION, FINELY DICED

---

1. Drain the tuna from the can and rinse.
2. Add tuna together with the rest of the ingredients in a serving bowl, mix thoroughly and cover with plastic wrap.
3. Serve right away or allow to marinate for as long as possible for more intense flavor.
4. Serve with a side salad or in a sandwich for lunch!

Per serving: Calories: 94; Fat: 1g; Carbohydrates: 11g; Phosphorus: 111mg; Potassium: 307mg ; Sodium: 144mg; Protein: 13g

SMOKED COD & PEA RISOTTO

SERVES 3 / PREP TIME: 5 MINUTES / COOK TIME: 45 MINUTES

A brilliant & classic combination.

- 1 TBSP EXTRA VIRGIN OLIVE OIL
- 1/2 WHITE ONION, FINELY DICED
- 1 CUP WHITE RICE
- 1 CUP HOMEMADE CHICKEN STOCK (p.52)
- 3 CUPS OF WATER
- 1/2 CUP OF FROZEN PEAS

- 4 OZ SKINLESS, BONELESS SMOKED COD FILLET
- 3 TBSP LOW FAT SOUR CREAM
- 1 TSP BLACK PEPPER
- 4 LEMON WEDGES
- 1 CUP OF ARUGULA

---

1. Heat the oil in a large pan on a medium heat.
2. Sauté the chopped onion for 5 minutes until soft before adding the rice and stirring.
3. Add half of the stock and water and stir slowly.
4. Slowly add the rest of the stock whilst continuously stirring for up to 20-30 minutes.
5. Stir in the peas to the risotto.
6. Place the fish on top of the rice, cover, and steam for 10 minutes.
7. Use your fork to break up the fish fillets and stir into the rice with the sour cream.
8. Sprinkle with freshly ground pepper to serve and a squeeze of fresh lemon.
9. Garnish with the lemon wedges and serve with the arugula on top.

Per serving: Calories: 228; Fat: 7g; Carbohydrates: 30g; Phosphorus: 197mg; Potassium: 290mg ; Sodium: 165mg; Protein: 11g

CUMIN CRAYFISH QUESADILLAS

SERVES 4 / PREP TIME: 5 MINUTES / COOK TIME: 15 MINUTES

Healthy homemade versions of the fast food favorite!

1/2 TSP PAPRIKA	4 TBSP SOUR CREAM
1/2 TSP GROUND CUMIN	FOR THE SALSA:
1/2 ORANGE	1/4 RED ONION, FINELY DICED
1/2 LEMON	1 JALAPEÑO, FINELY DICED
8 OZ RAW CRAYFISH	1/2 LEMON
4 WHITE TORTILLAS	1 TSP WHITE WINE VINEGAR

1. Prepare salsa by mixing salsa ingredients in a small bowl, cover and refrigerate until ready to eat.
2. Mix the paprika, cumin, orange and lemon juice together to prepare the marinade.
3. Add the crayfish to the marinade, cover and leave in refrigerator until ready to cook.
4. Heat a skillet over a medium heat and add the crayfish for 7-8 minutes or until cooked through.
5. Remove crayfish and place to one side.
6. Heat tortillas in the microwave for 30 seconds before adding salsa, crayfish, and sour cream.
7. Fold the tortilla in half, and add to skillet to heat through for 1 minute, turn and heat other side.
8. Repeat with the rest of the tortillas and serve.

Tip: Use lime instead of orange if you have been advised not to include oranges in your diet - check with your doctor if unsure.

Per serving: Calories: 181; Fat: 6g; Carbohydrates: 21g; Phosphorus: 210mg; Potassium: 326mg ; Sodium: 235mg; Protein: 11g

MEDITERRANEAN MONKFISH PAELLA

SERVES 2 / PREP TIME: 10 MINUTES / COOK TIME: 35 MINUTES

This paella dish will transport you straight to the Mediterranean Sea!

---

1 CUP WHITE/BROWN RICE (CHECK WHAT YOUR DIETITIAN RECOMMENDS)

3 CUPS OF WATER

2 TBSP EXTRA VIRGIN OLIVE OIL

1/2 WHITE ONION, DICED

2 GARLIC CLOVES, CRUSHED

1/4 TSP RED PEPPER FLAKES

3OZ MONKFISH FILLETS, DICED

1 TBSP PARSLEY, CRUSHED

1 LEMON, JUICE AND ZEST

1 LEMON – CUT INTO QUARTERS

---

1. Add the rice and 3 cups of water to a saucepan and boil on a high heat.
2. Once boiling, lower the heat, cover and simmer for 15 minutes.
3. Drain the rice and return to the heat for a further 3 minutes.
4. Place rice to one side.
5. In a skillet, heat the oil over a medium heat and then sauté the onion, garlic and red pepper flakes for 5 minutes until softened and then add the monkfish fillets.
6. Sauté for 6-9 minutes or until thoroughly cooked through and add the rice to the skillet.
7. Add the parsley, zest, and juice of 1 lemon, mixing well for a further 3-4 minutes.
8. Serve in a wide paella dish if possible or a large serving dish – scatter the lemon wedges around the edge and sprinkle with a little more fresh parsley.
9. Season with black pepper to taste.

Per serving: Calories: 286; Fat: 15g; Carbohydrates: 30g; Phosphorus: 200mg; Potassium: 236mg ; Sodium: 134mg; Protein: 8g

ORIENTAL SALMON BURGER

SERVES 3 / PREP TIME: 5 MINUTES / COOK TIME: 10 MINUTES

Healthy homemade version of the fast food favorite!

4OZ CANNED WILD SALMON, DRAINED

1 LARGE EGG WHITE, BEATEN

2 TBSP FRESH GINGER, MINCED

2 SCALLIONS, CHOPPED

1 TBSP COCONUT OIL

1 TSP WASABI POWDER

1/2 TSP HONEY

---

1. Combine the salmon, egg white, ginger, scallions and 1/2 tbsp. oil in a bowl, mixing well with your hands to form 4 patties.
2. In a separate bowl, add the wasabi powder with the honey and whisk until blended.
3. Heat 1/2 tbsp. oil over a medium heat in a skillet and cook the patties for 4 minutes per side until firm and browned.
4. Glaze the top of each patty with the wasabi mixture and cook for another 15 seconds before you serve.
5. Serve with your favorite side salad or vegetables for a healthy treat.

Per serving: Calories:135 ; Fat: 8g; Carbohydrates: 5g; Phosphorus: 149mg; Potassium: 263mg ; Sodium: 219mg; Protein: 12g

COCONUT POLLOCK AND BOK CHOY BROTH

SERVES 4 / PREP TIME: 5 MINUTES / COOK TIME: 25 MINUTES

Aromatic and spicy!

---

1 TSP BLACK PEPPER

1 CUP HOMEMADE CHICKEN STOCK (p.52)

1 CUP WATER

1 TSP COCONUT OIL

1 TSP FIVE-SPICE POWDER

1 TBSP OLIVE OIL

4 LEAVES OF BOK CHOY

1 TBSP GINGER, MINCED

2 CUPS NOODLES

1 GREEN ONION, THINLY SLICED

6 OZ POLLOCK FILLETS, SLICED

2 TSP CILANTRO, FINELY CHOPPED

---

1. In a bowl, combine pepper, 1/2 cup chicken stock, 1 cup water, coconut oil and spice blend.
2. Mix together and place to one side.
3. In a large saucepan, heat the oil over a medium heat and cook the bok choy and ginger for about 2 minutes until the bok choy is green.
4. Add the rest of the reserved chicken stock and heat through.
5. Add the noodles and stir, bringing to a simmer.
6. Add the green onion and the fish and cook for 10-15 minutes until fish is tender.
7. Add the fish, noodles, and vegetables into serving bowls and pour the broth over the top.
8. Garnish with the cilantro and serve with chopsticks for real authenticity!

Top tip: This works with most types of white fish or even salmon so switch things up according to what's sustainable at the time of cooking!

Per serving: Calories: 178; Fat: 6g; Carbohydrates: 19g; Phosphorus: 125mg; Potassium: 348mg ; Sodium: 72mg; Protein: 12g

HALIBUT WITH BUTTERY LEMON AND PARSLEY SAUCE

SERVES 2 / PREP TIME: 5 MINUTES / COOK TIME: 15 MINUTES

A meaty fish that tastes delicious with the citrus burst of the lemon.

1/2 LEMON

1 TSP EXTRA VIRGIN OLIVE OIL

4 OZ HALIBUT STEAK

1 TBSP UNSALTED BUTTER

2 TBSP WHITE ALL-PURPOSE FLOUR

1/2 CUP WATER

PINCH OF BLACK PEPPER

1 TBSP FRESH PARSLEY, FINELY CHOPPED

---

1. Mix 1 tbsp. lemon juice and olive oil in a large zip-lock bag, add the halibut and allow to marinate for at least 5 minutes in the fridge.
2. Meanwhile, heat a non-stick skillet over a medium heat, before adding the halibut to the skillet and cooking for 5 minutes.
3. Turn the fish over before cooking for a further 4 minutes and place to one side.
4. To make the sauce, melt the butter in the skillet over a low heat.
5. Now add flour and stir.
6. Add the water and stir for 1 minute.
7. Mix in the black pepper, parsley and the rest of the lemon juice, stirring for 3 minutes until the sauce thickens.
8. Slice the halibut into strips.
9. Add the halibut back into the sauce and heat until piping hot throughout.
10. Serve with your favorite side salad or vegetables and enjoy.

Per serving: Calories: 233; Fat: 19g; Carbohydrates: 8g; Phosphorus: 143mg; Potassium: 138mg ; Sodium: 154mg; Protein: 7g

SHRIMP AND ASPARAGUS LINGUINI

SERVES 5 / PREP TIME: 5 MINUTES / COOK TIME: 25 MINUTES

A delicious low fat pasta dish!

---

2 CUPS LINGUINI

6 ASPARAGUS STEMS

1 TBSP EXTRA VIRGIN OLIVE OIL

2 TBSP FRESH PARSLEY, CHOPPED

2 TBSP FRESH BASIL, CHOPPED

6 OZ COOKED SHRIMP

2 GARLIC CLOVES, MINCED

---

1. Preheat the oven to 350°f/170°c/Gas Mark 4.
2. Boil linguini for 15-20 minutes or according to package guidelines.
3. Meanwhile, add the asparagus stems to a baking sheet and drizzle with olive oil before baking for 7 to 8 minutes.
4. Remove from oven and transfer to a separate plate.
5. Once cool, cut asparagus into medium-sized pieces.
6. Heat skillet on a medium to high heat and add the herbs, shrimp, and garlic and stir until piping hot.
7. Add asparagus to the skillet.
8. Drain linguine and add to the skillet, using tongs to toss mixture through the linguine.
9. Drizzle with a little more olive oil to serve.

Per serving: Calories: 147; Fat: 4g; Carbohydrates: 19g; Phosphorus: 120 mg; Potassium: 156mg ; Sodium: 285mg; Protein: 10g

BAKED GARLIC HALIBUT

SERVES 2 / PREP TIME: 5 MINUTES / COOK TIME: 15 MINUTES

Succulent and delightful, this meaty fish tastes superb with the garlic.

---

4 OZ HALIBUT FILLET (OR ANY OTHER WHITE FISH OF YOUR CHOICE)

1 TSP BLACK PEPPER

1 TBSP DIJON MUSTARD

3 WHOLE GARLIC CLOVES, PRESSED AND SKIN ON

4 LEMON WEDGES TO GARNISH

2 TBSP EXTRA VIRGIN OLIVE OIL

---

1. Preheat oven to 400°f/190°c/Gas Mark 5.
2. Rub the fish with the pepper and mustard on both sides and add to a lined baking dish.
3. Scatter the garlic cloves around the fish and drizzle with the oil.
4. Squeeze the lemon juice over the fish.
5. Bake for approximately 15 minutes until the fish is firm and well cooked.
6. Divide into two and serve with the juices for a delicious garlic feast.

Tip: Serve this with your preference of vegetables or salad.

Per serving: Calories: 168; Fat: 15g; Carbohydrates: 3g; Phosphorus: 137mg; Potassium: 131mg ; Sodium: 178mg; Protein: 7g

FILIPINO STYLE SHRIMP NOODLES

SERVES 4 / PREP TIME: 10 MINUTES / COOK TIME: 25 MINUTES

This is inspired by a dish called Pancit Palabok, without the need to deep fry, making it suitable for the renal diet.

---

5 OZ WHOLE SHRIMP

1/2 TBSP CANOLA OIL

1/2 ONION, FINELY SLICED

1 GARLIC CLOVE, MINCED

8 OZ RICE NOODLES

FOR THE SAUCE:

2 CUPS WATER

2 GARLIC CLOVES, MINCED

1/2 TBSP CANOLA OIL

1 LEMON

1 GREEN ONION, FINELY SLICED

---

1. Prepare your shrimps by de-veining, peeling and cutting off heads (place heads to one side).
2. To make the sauce:
3. Add the shrimp heads and water to a processor and blend until smooth.
4. Now sieve this mixture through a strainer and return the liquid to the processor, add the rest of the shrimps and blend until smooth.
5. Now heat a pan/wok over a medium to high heat and add oil, onions, and garlic, stirring for 5-6 minutes until lightly golden.
6. Add shrimp sauce and noodles before turning down the heat and simmering for 15 minutes.
7. Slice the lemon.
8. Serve in bowls with sliced green onions and lemon wedges to garnish.

Per serving: Calories: 278; Fat: 4g; Carbohydrates:50g; Phosphorus: 122mg; Potassium: 79mg ; Sodium: 329mg; Protein: 8g

SWEET AND SOUR SHRIMP

SERVES 2 / PREP TIME: 10 MINUTES / COOK TIME: 20 MINUTES

A healthy version of the takeaway classic!

---

1 CELERY STALK, FINELY DICED

3 GREEN ONIONS, FINELY DICED

1 RED BELL PEPPER, FINELY DICED

1/2 CUP CANNED, SLICED WATER CHESTNUTS (NO ADDED SALT OR SUGAR)

4 WHOLE SHRIMPS

1 TBSP CANOLA OIL

FOR THE SWEET AND SOUR SAUCE:

1 TBSP RED CHILI FLAKES

2 TBSP LEMON JUICE

1/2 CUP PINEAPPLE, FINELY DICED

1/3 CUP WATER

1 TBSP FRESH GINGER, GRATED

---

1. Soak vegetables in warm water.
2. Meanwhile, prepare shrimp by slicing down the middle (not all the way through) and pulling apart to 'butterfly' - leave heads and tails on.
3. Heat the oil in a skillet on a medium to high heat.
4. Add the chestnuts, peppers, onion, and celery and sauté for 5 minutes.
5. Remove vegetables and place to one side.
6. Combine the sweet and sour sauce ingredients in a separate bowl.
7. Pour over your shrimp on a baking tray and allow to marinate for as long as possible.
8. Preheat the broiler to a medium heat.
9. Add the shrimp under the broiler and broil for 12-15 minutes or until cooked through.
10. Serve shrimp with the vegetables and enjoy.

Per serving: Calories: 153; Fat: 8g; Carbohydrates: 19g; Phosphorus: 65mg; Potassium: 346mg ; Sodium: 86mg; Protein: 5g

GREEN BEAN AND FENNEL TUNA SALAD

SERVES 3 / PREP TIME: 5 MINUTES / COOK TIME: 35 MINUTES

The aniseed taste of the fennel blends so well with the delicate green beans.

4OZ TUNA IN SPRING WATER

1 TSP CRUSHED BLACK PEPPERCORNS

1 TSP CRUSHED FENNEL SEEDS.

2 TBSP OLIVE OIL

1/2 CUP FENNEL BULB. TRIMMED

1/2 CUP WATER

1 LEMON. JUICED

1 CUP COOKED WHITE/BROWN RICE (CHECK WHAT YOUR DIETITIAN RECOMMENDS)

1 CUP FRESH GREEN BEANS. STEAMED

1 TSP FRESH PARSLEY. CHOPPED

1. Mix tuna with peppercorns and fennel seeds and rest for 10 minutes.
2. Heat the oil on a medium heat and sauté the fennel bulb slices for 5-6 minutes or until light brown.
3. Add the water to the pan and cook for 10 minutes until fennel is tender.
4. Stir in the lemon juice and lower heat to a simmer for another 5 minutes until liquid reduces.
5. Remove the fennel from the pan and slice.
6. Into an ovenproof dish add tuna mix with sliced fennel layered over the top and place under a broiler on a medium to high heat.
7. Broil for 5-6 minutes until top is crispy and brown.
8. Serve with rice & green beans. Garnish with the parsley.

Per serving: Calories: 216; Fat: 10g; Carbohydrates: 23g; Phosphorus: 141mg; Potassium: 348mg ; Sodium: 120mg; Protein: 10g

POLLOCK CHOWDER

SERVES 4 / PREP TIME: 5 MINUTES / COOK TIME: 1 HOUR

A traditional chowder dish, suitable for the renal diet.

---

6 CUPS WATER

6 OZ POLLOCK FILLET

1 TBSP OLIVE OIL

1 ONION, CHOPPED

1 STALK CELERY, CHOPPED

1 CAN OF CHOPPED TOMATOES (NO ADDED SALT OR SUGAR) - IF AVOIDING TOMATOES, USE A STOCK AS AN ALTERNATIVE

1 TBSP THYME, FINELY CHOPPED

1 TSP CAYENNE PEPPER

1 TSP BLACK PEPPER

2 BAY LEAVES

---

1. Boil the water in a small pan on a medium to high heat, and then add pollock fillet and simmer for 45 minutes.
2. Next, heat the oil in a pan on a medium heat and sauté the onion and the celery until browned.
3. Add the tomatoes, spices, and herbs and simmer for another minute or so.
4. Add the drained pollock fillets to the tomato sauce and simmer for a further 10 minutes.
5. Serve hot in individual serving bowls.

Per serving: Calories: 130; Fat: 8g; Carbohydrates: 9g; Phosphorus: 127mg; Potassium: 360mg ; Sodium: 40mg; Protein: 7g

PAN-SEARED HONEY COATED SALMON ON BABY ARUGULA

SERVES 2 / PREP TIME: 15 MINUTES / COOK TIME: 15 MINUTES

Rich in omega-3 and iron, this sweet and savory salmon dish is a winner.

---

3 OZ SKINLESS SALMON FILLET

2 TBSP EXTRA VIRGIN OLIVE OIL

1 TSP CHILI POWDER

1 TBSP HONEY

1/2 FRESH LIME, JUICED

A PINCH OF BLACK PEPPER TO TASTE

FOR THE SALAD:

1 CUPS BABY ARUGULA LEAVES

1/2 CUP SLIVERED RED ONION

1 TBSP OLIVE OIL

1 TBSP BALSAMIC VINEGAR

---

1. In a bowl, marinate the salmon with 1 tbsp. olive oil, lime juice, chili, honey and pepper and leave for at least 15 minutes (up to an hour).
2. Heat 1 tbsp. oil in a skillet over a medium heat and cook the salmon skin-side down for 6-7 minutes on each side or until thoroughly cooked through.
3. Toss the arugula and onions with oil and vinegar in a separate bowl.
4. Divide the salmon into two and serve on a bed of salad.

Per serving: Calories: 315; Fat: 22g; Carbohydrates: 18g; Phosphorus: 155mg; Potassium: 365mg ; Sodium: 234mg; Protein: 12g

SIMPLY SPICED
BAKED TROUT

SERVES 2 / PREP TIME: 5 MINUTES / COOK TIME: 15 MINUTES

Transports you straight to the water!

---

1 TBSP OLIVE OIL	4 OZ TROUT FILLET
1/2 TSP PAPRIKA	1 LEMON, HALVED
1 TSP CAYENNE PEPPER	1 GARLIC CLOVE

---

1. Preheat oven to 350° F/180°c/Gas Mark 4.
2. Whisk together the oil and spices in a small bowl.
3. Wash and pat dry the trout before coating both sides with oil and spices.
4. Add to a shallow baking dish with the lemon halves and garlic clove.
5. Bake uncovered for 20 to 30 minutes or until thoroughly cooked through and flaky.
6. Divide into two and serve with your choice of salad for a delicious Summer time supper!

Per serving: Calories: 184; Fat: 15g; Carbohydrates: 3g; Phosphorus: 130mg; Potassium: 230mg ; Sodium: 37mg; Protein: 11g

VEGETARIAN

VEGAN LASAGNA

SERVES 3 / PREP TIME: 10 MINUTES / COOK TIME: 1 HOUR

Just as scrumptious as its meaty friend!

1/2 PACK OF SOFT TOFU

1 GARLIC CLOVE, CRUSHED

4 TBSP OF RICE MILK (UNENRICHED)

2 TBSP OF FRESH BASIL, CHOPPED

1 LEMON, JUICED

A PINCH OF BLACK PEPPER TO TASTE

1/2 CUP BABY SPINACH

1 ZUCCHINI , SLICED

1 RED BELL PEPPER, SLICED

1 EGGPLANT, SLICED

---

1. Preheat oven to 325°F/170 °C/Gas Mark 3 and soak vegetables in warm water prior to cooking.
2. In a blender, process the tofu, garlic, milk, basil, lemon juice and pepper until smooth.
3. Toss in the spinach and zucchini for the last 30 seconds.
4. Layer the bottom of the dish with 1/3 the eggplant slices and 1/3 red pepper slices and then cover with 1/3 of the tofu sauce.
5. Repeat for a second layer.
6. Repeat for a third layer.
7. Bake in the oven for 1 hour or until the vegetables are soft through to the center (use your knife to test the middle).
8. Finish under the broiler until golden and bubbly.
9. Divide into portions and serve with a sprinkle of black pepper to taste.

Per serving: Calories: 91; Fat: 3g; Carbohydrates: 12g; Phosphorus: 110mg; Potassium: 368mg ; Sodium: 21mg; Protein: 6g

HOMEMADE RATATOUILLE

SERVES 2 / PREP TIME: 10 MINUTES / COOK TIME: 1-2 HOURS

Brimming with goodness and tasty flavor!

1 RED CHILI PEPPER, DICED

2 TBSP EXTRA VIRGIN OLIVE OIL

4 GARLIC CLOVES, MINCED

1 TBSP FRESH BASIL

1 TBSP FRESH OREGANO

1 TBSP FRESH ROSEMARY

1 TBSP FRESH THYME

1 TBSP FRESH SAGE

1 TBSP BLACK PEPPER

1 MEDIUM CARROT, DICED

1 CUP ONIONS, DICED

1 CUP ZUCCHINI, DICED

1 CUP SPAGHETTI SQUASH, DICED

2 CUPS EGGPLANT, DICED

1 CAN CHOPPED TOMATOES (NO ADDED SUGAR OR SALT)

1. Soak all vegetables in warm water prior to use.
2. Add the olive oil to a large skillet over a high heat.
3. Now add the garlic, herbs, black pepper and carrots.
4. Sauté for 5 minutes before adding the rest of the fresh vegetables and sautéing for 10-15 minutes.
5. Add the chopped tomatoes and stir.
6. Cover and simmer on a low heat for 1-2 hours, checking every so often to ensure the liquid doesn't dry out. Top up with water occasionally to prevent from drying up.
7. The sauce should reduce and be dark in color when ready and the vegetables will be extremely tender.

Per serving: Calories: 99; Fat: 5g; Carbohydrates: 14g; Phosphorus: 53mg; Potassium: 364mg; Sodium: 18mg; Protein: 2g

SUMMER BURGERS WITH CUCUMBER AND CHILI SALSA

SERVES 1 / PREP TIME: 5 MINUTES / COOK TIME: 15 MINUTES

These are wonderful in the summer and all year round for that matter!

EXTRA FIRM TEMPEH (1 PACK)	1/2 LIME, JUICED
1 TBSP EXTRA VIRGIN OLIVE OIL	1/2 RED ONION, FINELY DICED
1 TSP DRIED OREGANO	1 RED BELL PEPPER, DICED
1/2 CUCUMBER, FINELY DICED	1/2 CUP BABY SPINACH
1/4 RED CHILI, FINELY DICED	1 BUN (OPTIONAL)

1. Marinate the tempeh in 1/2 tbsp. oil and oregano combined.
2. Soak vegetables in warm water and heat the broiler on a medium to high heat.
3. Prepare your cucumber salsa by mixing the cucumber with the red chili and lime juice.
4. Heat 1/2 tbsp. olive oil in a skillet over a medium heat.
5. Sauté the onion in the skillet for 6-7 minutes or until caramelized.
6. Stir in the pepper and baby spinach for a further 3-4 minutes.
7. Place to one side.
8. Broil the tempeh on a lined oven-proof dish for 4 minutes on each side.
9. Add the tempeh to the bun and top with caramelized onion, spinach and diced peppers.
10. Serve immediately while hot with the cucumber salsa.

Per serving: Calories: 247; Fat: 13g; Carbohydrates: 25g; Phosphorus: 163mg; Potassium: 382mg ; Sodium: 151mg; Protein: 11g

OVEN-BAKED SPAGHETTI SQUASH

SERVES 4 / PREP TIME: 10 MINUTES / COOK TIME: 50 MINUTES

Autumnal and awesome!

1 PACK OF SOFT TOFU

1 TBSP COCONUT OIL

2 CLOVES GARLIC, MINCED

1 SPAGHETTI SQUASH, HALVED AND DESEEDED

1/2 CUP OF WATER

1 TBSP EXTRA VIRGIN OLIVE OIL

1. Get a medium-sized bowl and toss together the tofu, coconut oil and garlic.
2. Marinate and set aside for at least 30 minutes.
3. When ready to cook, preheat the oven to 375°F/190 °C/Gas Mark 5.
4. Grab a large baking dish and arrange the squash halves with the cut side down.
5. Pour half a cup of water into the dish.
6. Bake for around 45 minutes or until tender and remove the dish from the oven.
7. Turn the squash over and allow to cool.
8. Heat the oil on a medium heat in a skillet.
9. Add the tofu and cook for 8 minutes or until golden brown, occasionally stirring.
10. Remove and set aside.
11. Once cool, use your fork to scrape the spaghetti squash strands onto a serving dish.
12. Top with the tofu to serve.

Per serving: Calories: 154; Fat: 11g; Carbohydrates: 10g; Phosphorus: 118mg; Potassium: 370mg ; Sodium: 27mg; Protein: 8g

SPICED PEPPER CASSEROLE AND CRISPY TORTILLAS

SERVES 3 / PREP TIME: 10 MINUTES / COOK TIME: 40 MINUTES

A Mexican inspired dish.

---

1 CUP RED ONION, CHOPPED

1/2 ORANGE BELL PEPPER, CHOPPED

1/2 GREEN BELL PEPPER, CHOPPED

1 RED BELL PEPPER, CHOPPED

1 TBSP EXTRA VIRGIN OLIVE OIL

1 TSP BLACK PEPPER

1 TSP CHILI POWDER

1 TSP OREGANO, FRESH OR DRIED

1/2 CUP WATER

2 WHITE TORTILLAS

---

1. Soak the vegetables in warm water prior to cooking.
2. Heat the oil in a pot over a medium to high heat and add the red onion for 5 minutes.
3. Season with herbs and spices before adding in peppers and stirring for 5 minutes.
4. Add water, cover and simmer for 25-30 minutes.
5. Meanwhile, preheat the oven to its highest temperature.
6. Slice the tortillas into eighths and place on a baking tray in the oven for 5-10 minutes until crispy and golden.
7. Remove and allow to cool (they will go hard and crunchy like corn chips).
8. Serve the pepper casserole with the corn chips on the side and a salsa or dip of your choice.

Per serving: Calories: 130; Fat: 5g; Carbohydrates: 20g; Phosphorus: 92mg; Potassium: 292mg ; Sodium: 47g; Protein: 3g

BRILLIANT BEETROOT AND BRIE SALAD

SERVES 2 / PREP TIME: 5 MINUTES / COOK TIME: 8 MINUTES

A delightfully refreshing salad or light Summer's Evening meal.

---

2 TBSP EXTRA VIRGIN OLIVE OIL

1 ORANGE, JUICED

1 TSP DIJON MUSTARD

1 TBSP DILL, FINELY CHOPPED (FRESH OR DRIED)

1 CUP ROMAINE LETTUCE

1/2 CUP CANNED DICED BEETS (NO ADDED SALT OR SUGAR)

1 OZ BRIE

1 TSP BLACK PEPPER

---

1. Mix the oil, orange juice, mustard and chopped dill together in a salad bowl.
2. Add the romaine lettuce and toss to coat.
3. Serve the salad with the beetroot and brie cheese crumbled over the top.
4. Season with black pepper.

Tip: Use lime instead of orange if you have been advised not to include oranges in your diet - check with your doctor if unsure.

Per serving: Calories: 212; Fat: 18g; Carbohydrates:10g; Phosphorus: 51mg; Potassium: 236mg ; Sodium: 137mg; Protein: 4g

STIR FRIED PURPLE SPROUTING BROCCOLI AND BEAN SPROUTS

SERVES 2 / PREP TIME: 5 MINUTES / COOK TIME: 10 MINUTES

So simple yet so scrumptious!

---

1 CUP SPROUTING BROCCOLI OR CHINESE BROCCOLI

1/4 CUP BEAN SPROUTS

1 TBSP COCONUT OIL

2 CLOVES GARLIC, MINCED

1 TSP CHINESE 5 SPICE

1 THUMB SIZED PIECE FRESH GINGER, MINCED

1 TBSP RICE WINE VINEGAR

---

1. Soak vegetables in warm water prior to cooking.
2. Heat the oil in a skillet or wok on a high heat and add the garlic, spices, and ginger.
3. Cook for 1 minute.
4. Add the vegetables and rice wine vinegar to the skillet and sauté for a further 8-10 minutes.
5. Serve with cooked noodles or rice.

Per serving: Calories: 97; Fat: 7g; Carbohydrates: 8g; Phosphorus: 63mg; Potassium: 262mg ; Sodium: 55mg; Protein: 2g

SWEETCORN FRITTATA

SERVES 3 / PREP TIME: 5 MINUTES / COOK TIME: 25 MINUTES

Delicious with a side of seasonal greens.

---

6 EGG WHITES

1/2 CUP COCONUT MILK

1 TBSP COCONUT OIL

1 CUP FRESH OR FROZEN CORN

1 TSP BLACK PEPPER

---

1. Preheat the broiler to a medium heat.
2. Whisk the egg whites and coconut milk in a bowl.
3. Over a medium heat, add the coconut oil in an ovenproof (steel) frying pan.
4. When melted, add the corn and sauté for 5 minutes.
5. Add the egg mix to the pan and continue to cook on lowest heat for 7 minutes until light and bubbly.
6. Finish the frittata in its pan under the broiler for a further 5 -10 minutes or until crispy on the top and cooked through.
7. Slice and serve hot or allow to cool and serve chilled from the fridge!

Tip: Check with your doctor or dietitian as to whether you can still have coconut milk. Alternatively use a non-dairy milk such as almond.

Per serving: Calories: 96; Fat: 2g; Carbohydrates: 13g; Phosphorus: 52mg; Potassium: 223mg ; Sodium: 219mg; Protein: 9g

VEGETABLE AND APRICOT TAGINE

SERVES 2 / PREP TIME: 5 MINUTES / COOK TIME: 35 MINUTES

A vegetarian take on the Moroccan classic.

2 TBSP COCONUT OIL	1/2 CUP CARROTS, PEELED AND DICED
1/2 ONION, DICED	1 RED BELL PEPPER, DICED
1 TURNIP, PEELED AND DICED	1/2 CAN APRICOTS, JUICES DRAINED
2 CLOVES OF GARLIC	1 1/2 CUPS LOW SALT VEGETABLE STOCK
1 TSP GROUND CUMIN	1 1/2 CUPS OF WATER
1/2 TSP GROUND GINGER	2 TBSP LEMON JUICE
1/2 TSP GROUND CINNAMON	1/4 CUP CILANTRO, ROUGHLY CHOPPED
1/4 TSP CAYENNE PEPPER	

1. Soak the vegetables in warm water.
2. In a large pot, heat the oil on a medium high heat before sautéing the onion for 4-5 minutes until soft.
3. Add the turnip and cook for 10 minutes or until golden brown.
4. Add the garlic, cumin, ginger, cinnamon, and cayenne pepper, cooking for a further 3 minutes.
5. Add the carrots, red pepper, apricots, stock, and water to the pot and then bring to the boil.
6. Turn the heat down to a medium heat, cover and simmer for 20 minutes.
7. Add the lemon juice towards the end of cooking.
8. Garnish with the cilantro.

Tip: You can add potatoes or sweet potatoes to this dish: simply boil twice prior to cooking in order to lower the potassium.

Per serving: Calories: 173 ; Fat: 10g; Carbohydrates: 20g; Phosphorus: 78mg; Potassium: 391mg ; Sodium: 64mg; Protein: 4g

WILD GARLIC AND GREEN BEAN PESTO PASTA

SERVES 4 / PREP TIME: 5 MINUTES / COOK TIME: 20 MINUTES

Fresh and simple to make.

---

2 CUP FRESH WHITE PENNE PASTA

1/2 CUP FRESH BASIL, WASHED

1/2 CUP FRESH SPINACH/ARUGULA, WASHED

1/4 CUP EXTRA VIRGIN OLIVE OIL

1/4 CUP OF WILD GARLIC LEAVES (2 GARLIC CLOVES AS ALTERNATIVE)

1 LEMON, JUICED

2 CUP FRESH GREEN BEANS, TRIMMED AND SOAKED IN WARM WATER

1 TSP BLACK PEPPER

---

1. Bring a pan of water to the boil and add pasta, cooking for 15-20 minutes or according to package directions.
2. Meanwhile, blend all ingredients (minus green beans) in a food processor or a blender to reach required texture - chunky for a rustic feel or smooth as a dressing.
3. Add the green beans to steam over the pot of pasta for the last 10 minutes.
4. Drain pasta and stir through the pesto and green beans.
5. Serve with a sprinkle of black pepper to taste!

Per serving: Calories: 262; Fat: 14g; Carbohydrates: 29g; Phosphorus: 68mg; Potassium: 183mg ; Sodium: 5mg; Protein: 6g

CAULIFLOWER BHAJEES

SERVES 4 / PREP TIME: 5 MINUTES / COOK TIME: 8 MINUTES

A spicy Indian inspired treat.

---

2 CUPS CAULIFLOWER, FROZEN

4 EGG WHITES

1/2 CUP ONION, FINELY DICED

1 TSP CURRY POWDER

1 TBSP FRESH CILANTRO

2 TBSP ALL-PURPOSE WHITE FLOUR

1 TSP BLACK PEPPER

1 TBSP COCONUT OIL

---

1. Soak vegetables in warm water prior to cooking.
2. Steam cauliflower over a pan of boiling water for 10 minutes.
3. Blend eggs and onion in a food processor before adding cooked cauliflower, spices, cilantro, flour and pepper and blast in the processor for 30 seconds.
4. Heat a skillet over a high heat and add oil.
5. Pour tablespoon portions of the cauliflower mixture into the pan and brown on each side for 3-4 minutes or until crispy.
6. Enjoy hot with a crunchy side salad or seasonal greens.

Per serving: Calories: 174 ; Fat: 11g; Carbohydrates: 12g; Phosphorus: 101mg; Potassium: 288mg ; Sodium: 172mg; Protein: 7g

CRUNCHY TOFU STIR FRY

SERVES 3 / PREP TIME: 10 MINUTES / COOK TIME: 20 MINUTES

Easy yet scrumptious mid-week meal.

1/2 CUP SOFT TOFU

1 TBSP CORNSTARCH

2 EGG WHITES

1/2 CUP UNSEASONED WHITE BREAD CRUMBS

1 TBSP CANOLA OIL

1 RED BELL PEPPER, DICED

1 CUP FRESH BROCCOLI FLORETS

1 GARLIC CLOVE, MINCED

1 TSP BROWN SUGAR

1 TBSP FRESH LIME JUICE

1 TSP BLACK PEPPER

1 CUP COOKED WHITE RICE

---

1. Cut the tofu into cubes and soak the vegetables in warm water.
2. Place the cornstarch, egg whites and breadcrumbs each in their own separate bowls or serving dishes.
3. Dip the tofu cubes into each bowl consecutively.
4. Heat a skillet on a medium to high heat and add the oil.
5. Once hot, add the coated tofu to the skillet and cook for 7-8 minutes or until golden brown.
6. Remove and place to one side.
7. Add the bell pepper and broccoli and cook for 7-8 minutes or until crisp.
8. Add tofu back into the skillet and toss with the vegetables, sugar and fresh lime juice.
9. Sprinkle with black pepper and cooked rice.

Per serving: Calories: 261; Fat: 8g; Carbohydrates: 39g; Phosphorus: 167mg; Potassium: 359mg ; Sodium: 231mg; Protein: 11g

HOMEMADE CAULIFLOWER COUSCOUS AND BEETROOT SALSA

SERVES 4 / PREP TIME:10 MINUTES / COOK TIME: NA

This brilliantly vibrant couscous tastes delicious on a Summer's day!

---

1 LARGE HEAD CAULIFLOWER

1/2 CUCUMBER, PEELED AND DICED

1/4 CUP CANNED BEETROOT, DICED

1/2 CUP FRESH PARSLEY

1/2 CUP FRESH BASIL

1 LEMON

1 TSP BLACK PEPPER

---

1. Wash your cauliflower and soak in warm water prior to cooking.
2. When ready to serve, remove from warm water and allow to cool in the fridge.
3. Now grate the cauliflower head using the larger holes on a cheese grater to make your cauliflower couscous.
4. Add into a large serving dish and add cucumber, beetroot, freshly torn herbs and the juice of 1 lemon.
5. Toss with salad tongs and sprinkle with black pepper to serve.

Per serving: Calories: 35 ; Fat: 1g; Carbohydrates: 7g; Phosphorus: 44mg; Potassium: 255mg ; Sodium: 24mg; Protein: 2g

MIGHTY SCOTCH EGGS

SERVES 4 / PREP TIME: 10 MINUTES / COOK TIME: 15 MINUTES

Please consult with your dietitian as to whether you can have whole eggs as part of your diet. If so, these are such a tasty and handy snack!

---

5 LARGE EGGS

2 TBSP EXTRA VIRGIN OLIVE OIL

1/2 ONION, FINELY DICED

2 TBSP FRESH PARSLEY, FINELY CHOPPED

1 CUP WHITE BREADCRUMBS

1 TBSP ALL PURPOSE WHITE FLOUR

---

1. Put 4 eggs into a pan of cold water and bring to the boil.
2. Once boiling, carefully add the eggs to the pan for 6 minutes before draining and running under cold water.
3. Peel eggs and set aside.
4. Heat 1 tbsp oil in a pan on a medium to high heat and add the onion, sautéing for 5-6 minutes.
5. Remove onions and allow to cool in a separate bowl for a few minutes before beating in the 5th egg and parsley and breadcrumbs.
6. Spread out a sheet of plastic wrap.
7. Divide mixture into 4 and place 1 portion into the center of the wrap.
8. Dust 1 egg with flour and place in the center of the mixture.
9. Use the wrap to wrap the mixture around the egg, coating all the way around.
10. Repeat with the remaining mixture and eggs.
11. If the mixture does not stick, try adding a little more flour/egg to the mixture.
12. If it is too runny then you will need to add more breadcrumbs.
13. Add 1 tbsp oil to a pan and add the eggs to brown on all sides, cooking for 7-8 minutes in total or until crispy.
14. These taste great alone as a snack or with your favorite veggies as a more filling meal.

Per serving: Calories: 274; Fat: 14g; Carbohydrates: 24g; Phosphorus: 180mg; Potassium: 195mg ; Sodium: 277mg; Protein: 12g

MIDDLE EASTERN EGGPLANT

SERVES 2 / PREP TIME:10 MINUTES / COOK TIME:40 MINUTES

Lusciously spiced!

---

1 EGGPLANT

1/2 RED ONION, FINELY DICED

1 GARLIC CLOVE, MINCED

1 TBSP FRESH OR DRIED PARSLEY

1 TSP FRESH OR DRIED OREGANO

1 TSP CUMIN

1 TBSP EXTRA VIRGIN OLIVE OIL

1/2 LEMON, JUICED

1 TSP BLACK PEPPER

1 CUP ARUGULA

---

1. Soak vegetables in warm water prior to cooking.
2. Preheat the oven to 350°f/170°c/Gas Mark 4.
3. Cut eggplant in half lengthways and add face up to a lightly oiled baking tray - add to the oven for 20 minutes or until starting to soften.
4. Meanwhile, mix the onion, garlic, herbs, spices, olive oil, lemon juice and black pepper in a separate bowl. Place to one side.
5. Remove the eggplant from the oven and very carefully scoop out the flesh from the insides of the eggplant to create a shallow well in each half. Combine the flesh with the onion mix and whiz up in a blender for 30 seconds to combine (alternatively, chop the flesh into very small pieces and mix by hand.)
6. Now spoon the mixture back into the eggplant halves and return to the oven for 15-20 minutes or until bubbling hot.
7. Enjoy hot with a side of arugula.

Per serving: Calories: 132 ; Fat: 7g; Carbohydrates: 17g; Phosphorus: 51mg; Potassium: 313mg ; Sodium: 11mg; Protein: 2g

SPANISH PAPRIKA POTATOES

SERVES 3 / PREP TIME: 5 MINUTES / COOK TIME: 30 MINUTES

Transport yourself to the continent and taste the sunshine!

2 SWEET POTATOES	1/2 LEMON
1 TBSP EXTRA VIRGIN OLIVE OIL	1 TBSP LOW FAT SOUR CREAM
1 TBSP SMOKED PAPRIKA	
1 TBSP FRESHLY CHOPPED PARSLEY	

1. Peel and cut the potatoes into 1 inch cubes.
2. Place in a pan of boiling water for 10 minutes before draining water completely and bringing a new pan of water to the boil.
3. Add potatoes to the pan again for 10 minutes.
4. Meanwhile, add the oil to a skillet on a medium to high heat.
5. Add the potatoes and sprinkle over the paprika; sauté for 15 minutes.
6. Serve in a dish with the fresh herbs, lemon juice and a dollop of sour cream on the top.

Per serving: Calories: 92; Fat: 5g; Carbohydrates: 11g; Phosphorus: 34g; Potassium: 271mg ; Sodium: 21mg; Protein: 1g

EGGPLANT FRENCH FRIES WITH CARROT AND ORANGE HUMMUS

SERVES 3 / PREP TIME: 5 MINUTES / COOK TIME: 30 MINUTES

A tastebud sensation!

FOR THE FRIES:

1 MEDIUM EGGPLANT

2 EGG WHITES

1 CUP RICE MILK (UNENRICHED)

3/4 CUP CORNSTARCH

3/4 CUP DRY UNSEASONED WHITE BREAD CRUMBS

1/4 CUP CANOLA OIL

FOR THE HUMMUS:

3 TBSP EXTRA VIRGIN OLIVE OIL

1 TSP CLEAR HONEY

1 CUP CARROTS, PEELED AND DICED

1 GARLIC CLOVE, MINCED

1/2 TSP CUMIN SEEDS

1/2 TSP CILANTRO SEEDS

1/2 ORANGE

1 TSP BLACK PEPPER

1. Prepare your hummus by adding all the hummus ingredients to a food processor or blender and whizzing up until smooth.
2. Place to one side.
3. Peel and slice the eggplant into fries.
4. Whisk the eggs and milk in a medium-sized bowl.
5. In a separate shallow bowl, mix the cornstarch and breadcrumbs.
6. Add the oil to a skillet over a medium to high heat.
7. Dip the eggplant fries into the egg mixture, followed by the breadcrumb mixture.
8. Add to the piping hot oil and cook for 3 minutes until crispy.
9. Add to a plate with kitchen towel and serve with the hummus.

Tip: Use lime instead of orange if you have been advised not to include oranges in your diet - check with your doctor if unsure.

Per serving: Calories: 342 ; Fat: 12g; Carbohydrates: 51g; Phosphorus: 90mg; Potassium: 352mg ; Sodium: 256mg; Protein: 7g

VEGETABLE PAELLA

SERVES 2 / PREP TIME: 10 MINUTES / COOK TIME: 25 MINUTES

Herby and fresh - amazing!

1/2 CUP ASPARAGUS, CHOPPED

1 CUP RED BELL PEPPER, CHOPPED

1/2 ZUCCHINI, CHOPPED

1/2 RED ONION, CHOPPED

1 CUP WHITE RICE

1 TBSP EXTRA VIRGIN OLIVE OIL

1 TSP OREGANO (DRIED)

1 TSP PARSLEY (DRIED)

1 TSP PAPRIKA

1/2 LEMON

1 CUP LOW-SALT VEGETABLE STOCK

---

1. Soak vegetables in warm water prior to cooking.
2. Add rice to a pot of cold water and cook for 15 minutes.
3. Drain the water, cover the pan and leave to one side.
4. Heat the oil in a skillet and add the asparagus, bell pepper, onion, and zucchini, sautéing for 5 minutes.
5. To the pan, add the rice, herb, spices, and juice of the lemon along with the vegetable stock.
6. Cover and turn heat right down and allow to simmer for 15-20 minutes.
7. Serve hot.

Per serving: Calories: 168; Fat: 6g; Carbohydrates: 26g; Phosphorus: 100mg; Potassium: 384mg ; Sodium: 33mg; Protein: 5g

CHARGRILLED CHILI & HONEY TURNIPS WITH ZUCCHINI PASTA

SERVES 2 / PREP TIME: 10 MINUTES / COOK TIME: 40 MINUTES

Gloriously healthy homemade pasta with a crunchy topping.

2 TURNIPS, PEELED AND CUT INTO FINE SHAVINGS

1 TSP CLEAR HONEY

1 TSP RED CHILI FLAKES

2 ZUCCHINIS, PEELED AND SLICED VERTICALLY TO MAKE NOODLES (USE A SPIRALIZER)

1 TBSP EXTRA VIRGIN OLIVE OIL

1/2 CUP ARUGULA

1/2 LEMON

1. Preheat the oven to 350°f/170°c/Gas Mark 4.
2. Soak the vegetables in warm water prior to cooking.
3. Spread the turnip slices over a baking tray and drizzle over honey before sprinkling with chili flakes.
4. Toss to coat.
5. Add to the oven for 35-40 minutes or until cooked through and slightly crispy.
6. Meanwhile, heat a pan of water on a high heat and bring to the boil.
7. Add the zucchini noodles and turn the heat down to simmer for 3-4 minutes.
8. Remove from the heat and place in a bowl of cold water immediately.
9. Serve zucchini noodles with turnip shavings and a drizzle of olive oil on top.
10. Mix the arugula with the lemon juice and serve on the side.
11. Enjoy!

Per serving: Calories: 85; Fat: 5g; Carbohydrates: 10g; Phosphorus: 62mg; Potassium: 336mg; Sodium: 9mg; Protein: 2g

VEGETARIAN CURRIED KEDGEREE

SERVES 4 / PREP TIME: 5 MINUTES / COOK TIME: 30 MINUTES

A vegetarian take on a classic dish. Tip: Leave the eggs out if they are restricted from your diet. Consult your doctor if unsure.

---

1 ONION, CUT INTO QUARTERS

1/2 EGGPLANT, CUT INTO QUARTERS

1 ZUCCHINI, CUT INTO QUARTERS

1/2 RED BELL PEPPER, CUT INTO QUARTERS

1 TBSP EXTRA VIRGIN OLIVE OIL

1 TSP CURRY POWDER

1 TSP BLACK PEPPER

1 CUP RICE, RINSED THOROUGHLY

2 EGGS

1 TBSP FRESH CHIVES, CHOPPED

---

1. Soak vegetables in warm water prior to serving and preheat the oven to 375°F/190°C/Gas Mark 5.
2. Add the vegetables to an oven dish and toss together.
3. Drizzle with oil and sprinkle with curry powder and pepper - toss to coat.
4. Bake in the oven for 30 minutes, stirring occasionally.
5. Meanwhile, add the rice to a pot of cold water and bring to the boil over a high heat.
6. Simmer for 10 minutes until rice has nearly soaked up all of the water.
7. Turn the heat to the lowest temperature and cover the pan for a further 5-10 minutes until light and fluffy.
8. Boil a separate pan of water and add the eggs for 7 minutes.
9. Run under the cold tap, crack and peel the eggs before cutting in half.
10. Toss the rice with the roasted vegetables and top with eggs and chopped chives.
11. Serve hot!

Per serving: Calories: 162; Fat: 6g; Carbohydrates: 24g; Phosphorus: 103mg; Potassium: 308mg ; Sodium: 79mg; Protein: 5g

BRIE, CHIVE AND SCALLION TART

SERVES 4 / PREP TIME: 10 MINUTES / COOK TIME: 50 MINUTES

A delicious spring treat.

FOR THE PASTRY:

1 CUP ALL PURPOSE WHITE FLOUR

1/2 CUP UNSALTED BUTTER, CUBED

1/4 CUP RICE MILK (UNENRICHED)

FOR THE FILLING:

1 EGG

1 EGG YOLK

1 CUP RICE MILK (UNENRICHED)

1 TSP BLACK PEPPER

2 STEMS OF SCALLION, CHOPPED

1/2 CUP BRIE

1 TBSP CHIVES, FINELY CHOPPED

APPROX. 10CM TART TIN

BAKING BEADS

FOIL

---

1. Sift the flour and add the butter by rubbing with fingers to create a breadcrumb texture.
2. Mix in the milk for the pastry slowly to bind and then knead on a work surface into a ball shape.
3. Wrap dough in plastic wrap and add to the fridge to cool.
4. Preheat the oven to 350°f/180°c/Gas Mark 4.
5. Lightly flour the work surface and use a rolling pin to roll the pastry to approx. 1cm thick.
6. Gently use your fingers to lift the pastry over the base of the tart tin.
7. Line the pastry with the foil followed by the baking beads and add to the oven for 15 minutes.
8. Now trim the edges of the pastry from around the pastry tin.
9. Remove beads and foil and score the pastry with a fork before adding back into the oven for a further 15 minutes or until starting to turn golden.
10. While the pastry is cooking prepare the filling by beating the egg, egg yolk and milk in a separate bowl and seasoning with pepper.
11. Add the chopped scallions, crumbled brie and chopped chives to this mixture and gently pour into the pastry base.
12. Bake in the oven for 35 minutes or until cooked through and golden.
13. Serve warm.

Per serving: Calories: 456 ; Fat:33g; Carbohydrates: 29g; Phosphorus: 147mg; Potassium: 198mg ; Sodium: 208mg; Protein: 11g

NORTH AFRICAN SPAGHETTI SQUASH CURRY

SERVES 3 / PREP TIME: 10 MINUTES / COOK TIME: 40 MINUTES

A hearty, chunky dish packed full with flavor.

- 1 TBSP EXTRA VIRGIN OLIVE OIL
- 1 ONION, DICED
- 1 TSP BLACK PEPPER
- 1 TSP TURMERIC
- 1 TSP CUMIN
- 1 TSP GINGER, GRATED
- 1 GARLIC CLOVE, CHOPPED

- 1/2 STALK CELERY, CHOPPED
- 1/2 CAN CHOPPED TOMATOES (NO ADDED SALT OR SUGAR)
- 1 CUP WATER
- 2 TBSP FRESH CILANTRO
- 1 CUP SPAGHETTI SQUASH

---

1. In a large pot, heat the oil over a medium to high heat.
2. Add the onions.
3. After 5 minutes, turn the heat down and sprinkle with pepper, turmeric, cumin and ginger.
4. Now add garlic and celery and continue to sauté for 5 minutes.
5. Add the tomatoes (use homemade stock in place of tomatoes if these are restricted from your diet) and water along with half the cilantro and simmer.
6. Meanwhile, prepare the squash by peeling and chopping into chunky cubes.
7. Add the squash to the pan and continue to cook for 30 minutes, stirring occasionally until soft.
8. Scatter with the rest of the cilantro to serve.

Per serving: Calories: 106; Fat: 5g; Carbohydrates: 15g; Phosphorus: 54mg; Potassium: 375mg ; Sodium: 27mg; Protein: 2g

OVEN BAKED RED PEPPER STEW

SERVES 3 / PREP TIME: 10 MINUTES / COOK TIME: 40 MINUTES

A hearty Winter's stew.

---

2 RED BELL PEPPERS, ROUGHLY CHOPPED

1/2 RED ONION, ROUGHLY CHOPPED

1 TBSP EXTRA VIRGIN OLIVE OIL

1 TSP PARSLEY

1 TSP CUMIN

1 GARLIC CLOVE, CRUSHED

1/2 CAN CHOPPED TOMATOES (NO ADDED SALT OR SUGAR)

1 TBSP BALSAMIC VINEGAR

1/2 CUP WATER

1 TSP BLACK PEPPER

2 EGGS (SKIP IF EGGS ARE RESTRICTED)

---

1. Soak vegetables in water prior to cooking and preheat the oven to 350°f/170°c/Gas Mark 4.
2. Grab an oven proof baking dish and add all of the ingredients (minus the eggs) stirring well.
3. Bake in the oven for 30-35 minutes or until vegetables are very soft (keep an eye on liquid throughout and top up with water to keep it from drying up).
4. Turn off the oven and heat up the broiler.
5. Remove the oven dish and crack both eggs over the top before placing under the broiler to broil for 6-7 minutes or until cooked through.
6. Portion up and serve hot with black pepper to taste.

Per serving: Calories: 128 ; Fat: 7g; Carbohydrates: 12g; Phosphorus: 94mg; Potassium: 363mg; Sodium: 116mg; Protein: 5g

MEDITERRANEAN VEGETABLE PIZZA

SERVES 4 / PREP TIME: 10 MINUTES / COOK TIME: 50 MINUTES

Healthy kidney pizza!

---

8 EGG WHITES

1/2 CUP FRESH CHOPPED BASIL

1 TBSP CHOPPED OREGANO

1/2 CUP OF CANNED CHOPPED TOMATOES (NO ADDED SALT OR SUGAR)

1 ZUCCHINI, PEELED AND SLICED

1/2 RED BELL PEPPER, SLICED

4 CRUSHED GARLIC CLOVES

1/2 RED ONION, PEELED AND SLICED

1 TBSP EXTRA VIRGIN OLIVE OIL

1/4 CUP BRIE

---

1. Preheat oven to 350°f/180°c/Gas Mark 4.
2. Whisk the eggs, basil, and oregano in a bowl and mix in the tomatoes.
3. Layer zucchini, pepper, garlic and onion slices in a round baking dish and drizzle with olive oil.
4. Roast in the oven for 15 minutes.
5. Pour the tomato and egg mixture over the vegetables in the baking dish.
6. Bake in the oven for 35-40 minutes, or until the center is cooked through (check with a knife).
7. Sprinkle crumbled brie over the top and place under the broiler to brown.
8. Enjoy warm or cooled in the fridge with your favorite side salad.

Per serving: Calories: 128; Fat: 6g; Carbohydrates: 9g; Phosphorus: 69mg; Potassium: 367mg ; Sodium: 273mg; Protein: 11g

SAVORY CHEESE AND ONION PANCAKES

SERVES 3 / PREP TIME: 5 MINUTES / COOK TIME: 10 MINUTES

Quick to prepare and delicious. Please avoid if eggs are restricted from your diet.

1/2 WHITE ONION, FINELY DICED

2 EGGS

1/2 CUP RICE MILK (UNENRICHED)

1/2 CUP WATER

1 TSP BLACK PEPPER

1 CUP WHITE ALL-PURPOSE FLOUR

1 TBSP EXTRA VIRGIN OLIVE OIL

1/4 CUP BRIE, CRUMBLED

1. Soak onion in warm water.
2. In a medium bowl add the eggs, milk, water, and pepper together until combined.
3. Add the flour to the mix and whisk into a smooth paste.
4. Melt a drizzle of oil in a skillet over a medium heat.
5. Add 1/3 pancake mixture to form a round pancake shape.
6. Cook for 4-5 minutes until the bottom is light brown and easily comes away from the pan with the spatula.
7. Flip and add 1/3 raw onion and 1/3 crumbled brie over the top before cooking for a further 4 minutes.
8. Fold and serve warm - the cheese should have melted and the onions will be warm but still crunchy.
9. Serve and repeat with the rest of the ingredients.

Per serving: Calories: 303; Fat: 11g; Carbohydrates: 38g; Phosphorus: 150mg; Potassium: 221mg ; Sodium: 199mg; Protein: 11g

SIDES, SALADS AND SOUPS

TARRAGON AND PEPPER PASTA SALAD

SERVES 4 / PREP TIME: 10 MINUTES / COOK TIME: 35 MINUTES

A lovely addition to a BBQ or a meal on its own.

---

2 CUPS WHITE PASTA

1 RED BELL PEPPER, FINELY DICED

1/2 CUCUMBER, FINELY DICED

1/4 RED ONION, FINELY SLICED

1 TSP BLACK PEPPER

2 TBSP EXTRA VIRGIN OLIVE OIL

1 TBSP DRIED TARRAGON

---

1. Bring a pan of water to the boil before adding pasta for 15-20 minutes or according to package directions.
2. Drain and allow pasta to cool before combining the rest of the raw ingredients and mixing well.
3. Serve right away or cover and refrigerate for 2-3 days.

Per serving: Calories: 156; Fat: 7g; Carbohydrates: 20g; Phosphorus: 46mg; Potassium: 147mg ; Sodium: 2mg; Protein: 4g

SPICED PUMPKIN PANCAKES

SERVES 2 / PREP TIME: 5 MINUTES / COOK TIME: 6 MINUTES

A great go-to made with your pantry essentials. Enjoy low sodium canned pumpkin in early stages of kidney disease and always check with your doctor.

1 CUP OF CANNED PUMPKIN, NO ADDED SALT OR SUGAR

2 TBSP WATER

3 EGG WHITES

1 TSP PAPRIKA

1 TSP CAYENNE PEPPER

1 TSP CINNAMON

1 TBSP COCONUT OIL

1. Blend the pumpkin flesh together with water to form a smooth pulp.
2. Now add the rest of the ingredients (minus the coconut oil) and mix well.
3. Heat coconut oil in a large skillet.
4. Pour the pumpkin mixture into the pan into individual rounded pancakes (go easy at first and pour your mixture into little circles, keep pouring whilst tilting the pan until you have a pancake to your desired shape).
5. Lift the mixture with a spatula and then flip. Cook for 3 minutes on either side.
6. Serve warm - they taste great with sweet or savory accompaniments.

Per serving: Calories: 125; Fat: 8g; Carbohydrates: 13g; Phosphorus: 55mg; Potassium: 355mg ; Sodium: 298mg; Protein: 5g

LEMON AND PARSLEY COLESLAW

SERVES 2 / PREP TIME: 15 MINUTES / COOK TIME: N/A

Lovely healthy side dish or snack.

1 CARROT, PEELED AND FINELY SLICED

1 CUP WHITE CABBAGE, PEELED AND FINELY SLICED

1 LEMON, JUICE AND ZEST

1 TBSP FRESH PARSLEY, FINELY CHOPPED

1 TBSP EXTRA VIRGIN OLIVE OIL

1. Soak vegetables in warm water for 5-10 minutes.
2. Drain and rinse with cold water.
3. Combine with the rest of the ingredients, cover and cool in refrigerator before serving.

Per serving: Calories: 89; Fat: 7g; Carbohydrates: 7g; Phosphorus: 25mg; Potassium: 208mg ; Sodium: 30mg; Protein: 1g

TURNIP CHIPS

SERVES 2 / PREP TIME: 5 MINUTES / COOK TIME: 50 MINUTES

A healthy kidney friendly snack.

---

1 TBSP EXTRA VIRGIN OLIVE OIL

2 TURNIPS, PEELED AND SLICED

1 TSP BLACK PEPPER

1 TSP OREGANO

1 TSP PAPRIKA

1 CLOVE MINCED GARLIC

---

1. Heat oven to 375°f/190°c/Gas Mark 5.
2. Grease a baking tray with the olive oil.
3. Add turnip slices in a thin layer.
4. Dust over herbs and spices with an extra drizzle of olive oil.
5. Bake for 40-50 minutes (turning half way through to ensure even crispiness!)

Per serving: Calories: 128; Fat: 7g; Carbohydrates: 16g; Phosphorus: 60mg; Potassium: 327mg ; Sodium: 14mg; Protein: 2g

SPICED GINGER AND CABBAGE SOUP

SERVES 4 / PREP TIME: 10 MINUTES / COOK TIME: 35 MINUTES

A real zingy soup – great for winter but can be served cooled in the Summer too!

2 TBSP OLIVE OIL	1 ONION, CHOPPED
1 TSP MUSTARD SEEDS, GROUND	ZEST AND JUICE OF 1 LIME
1 TSP CILANTRO SEEDS, GROUND	1 CUP LOW-SALT VEGETABLE STOCK
1 TSP CURRY POWDER	3 CUPS OF WATER
1 TBSP GINGER, MINCED	BLACK PEPPER TO TASTE
2 CUPS CABBAGE, THINLY SLICED	

1. In a pan on a medium heat, add the oil then the seeds and curry powder for 1 minute.
2. Add the ginger and cook for a further minute.
3. Then add the cabbage, onions and the lime juice, cooking for at least 2 minutes or until the vegetables are soft.
4. Add the stock and water and allow to boil before turning the heat down slightly and simmering for 30 minutes.
5. Allow to cool.
6. Put the mixture in a food processor and puree until smooth.
7. Serve with lime zest and black pepper.

Per serving: Calories: 118; Fat: 8g; Carbohydrates: 12g; Phosphorus: 70mg; Potassium: 322mg ; Sodium: 34mg; Protein: 3g

SPAGHETTI SQUASH SOUP

SERVES 4 / PREP TIME: 10 MINUTES / COOK TIME: 45 MINUTES

Winter warming soup.

---

1 TBSP CANOLA OIL

1 ONION, QUARTERED AND SLICED

2 LARGE GARLIC CLOVES, CHOPPED

3 CUPS HOMEMADE CHICKEN STOCK (p. 52)

3 CUPS OF WATER

2 CUPS SPAGHETTI SQUASH, PEELED AND CUBED

1 SPRIG OF THYME/1 TBSP DRIED THYME

1 TSP CHILI POWDER

---

1. Soak vegetables in warm water prior to cooking.
2. Heat oil in a large pan on a medium high heat before sweating the onions and garlic for 3-4 minutes.
3. Add the stock and water, and bring to a boil over a high heat before adding the squash.
4. Turn down heat and allow to simmer for 25-30 minutes.
5. Now add the rest of the ingredients and simmer for a further 15 minutes or until the squash is tender.
6. Serve hot!

Per serving: Calories: 103; Fat: 5g; Carbohydrates: 12g; Phosphorus: 83mg; Potassium: 319mg; Sodium: 99mg; Protein: 5g

SPICY PEPPER SOUP

Wonderfully satisfying!

---

2 1/2 TBSP OF EXTRA VIRGIN OLIVE OIL

1 RED ONION, CHOPPED

4 RED BELL PEPPERS, CHOPPED

2 GARLIC CLOVES, CHOPPED

2 HABANERO CHILIS WITH THE STEMS REMOVED AND CHOPPED

3 CUPS HOMEMADE CHICKEN STOCK (p. 52)

---

1. In a pan on a medium heat, add the oil then the onions and peppers, sweating for 5 minutes.
2. Add the garlic cloves and chilis and sauté for 3-4 minutes.
3. Add the stock and allow to boil before turning heat down slightly and simmering for 30 minutes.
4. Allow to cool.
5. Put the mixture in a food processor and puree until smooth.
6. Serve with black pepper.

Per serving: Calories: 152; Fat: 10g; Carbohydrates: 14g; Phosphorus: 92mg; Potassium: 400mg; Sodium: 58g; Protein: 5g

GREEN ONION & LEMON BULGUR SIDE

SERVES 2 / PREP TIME: 35 MINUTES / COOK TIME: NA

This is very simple to make and tastes great with chicken, fish or roasted vegetables.

---

1 BUNCH GREEN ONIONS, FINELY CHOPPED

1/2 CUP DRY BULGUR

1/4 CUP EXTRA VIRGIN OLIVE OIL

1 LEMON

3 TBSP FRESH PARSLEY

3 TBSP FRESH MINT

1 TSP BLACK PEPPER

---

1. Soak the onions in warm water.
2. Meanwhile, wash the bulgur before adding to a bowl.
3. Pour 1/2 cup boiling water over the bulgur, cover and leave to sit for 30 minutes.
4. Drain any excess liquid from the bulgur.
5. Drain the vegetables and add to the bulgur, mixing well.
6. Add olive oil, lemon juice, herbs, and pepper to the bulgur mixture.
7. Let salad set at room temperature for about an hour to absorb the lemon juice and olive oil before serving.
8. Refrigerate leftovers in an airtight container for 2-3 days.

Per serving: Calories: 375; Fat: 28g; Carbohydrates: 31g; Phosphorus: 72mg; Potassium: 219mg; Sodium: 14mg; Protein: 5g

ASIAN STYLE BROTH

SERVES 4 / PREP TIME: 5 MINUTES / COOK TIME: 20 MINUTES

Fresh and full of delicious Asian-infused flavors.

1 TBSP CILANTRO SEEDS

2 TBSP OLIVE OIL

1 WHITE ONION, CHOPPED

1 GARLIC CLOVE, MINCED

1 THUMB SIZE PIECE OF MINCED GINGER

1/2 CUP OF COCONUT MILK

1/2 CUP OF HOMEMADE CHICKEN STOCK (p. 52)

1 EGGPLANT, DICED

A HANDFUL OF FRESH BASIL LEAVES

1/2 CUP BABY SPINACH LEAVES

1 RED CHILI, FINELY CHOPPED

2 STEMS OF GREEN ONION, CHOPPED

1 FRESH LIME

1. Crush the cilantro seeds in a blender or pestle and mortar.
2. Mix in 1 tbsp. olive oil until a paste is formed.
3. Heat a large pan/wok with 1 tbsp. olive oil on a high heat.
4. Fry the onions, garlic, and ginger until soft but not crispy or browned.
5. Into the pan, add the spice paste from earlier along with the coconut milk and stir.
6. Slowly add the stock until a broth is formed.
7. Now add the eggplant and allow to simmer in the broth for 10-15 minutes.
8. Add the basil and spinach 2-3 minutes before the end of the cooking time.
9. Serve hot with the chili and green onion sprinkled over the top.
10. Squeeze lime juice over to finish.

Tip: Check with your doctor or dietitian as to whether you can still have coconut milk. Alternatively use a non-dairy milk such as almond.

Per serving: Calories: 185; Fat: 14g; Carbohydrates: 15g; Phosphorus: 76mg; Potassium: 340mg; Sodium: 21mg; Protein: 3g

CURRIED ONION AND CAULIFLOWER SOUP

SERVES 4 / PREP TIME: 10 MINUTES / COOK TIME: 40 MINUTES

A delicious lightly spiced soup.

2 TBSP COCONUT OIL	1 TSP CUMIN
1 ONION, PEELED AND CHOPPED	1 TSP TURMERIC
4 CLOVES GARLIC, MINCED	1 CUP HOMEMADE CHICKEN STOCK (p. 52)
1/2 CAULIFLOWER, CHOPPED	3 CUPS WATER
3 SLICES CELERY, CHOPPED	1 CUP LOW FAT COCONUT MILK

1. Heat the oil in a large pan over a medium to high heat.
2. Add the onions, garlic and cauliflower and sweat for 5-10 minutes (don't let them brown).
3. Add the celery and spices and cook for another 5 minutes.
4. Add the stock and water and bring to a boil before lowering heat and simmering for 15-20 minutes or until celery is soft.
5. Remove from heat and allow to cool before blending in a food processor or liquidizer (don't panic if you don't have one, you can enjoy this soup as a chunky soup!)
6. Return to the pan and add the coconut milk, warming through.
7. Serve with a sprinkle of black pepper.

Tip: Check with your doctor or dietitian as to whether you can still have coconut milk. Alternatively use a non-dairy milk such as almond.

Per serving: Calories: 184; Fat: 15g; Carbohydrates: 13g; Phosphorus: 94mg; Potassium: 400mg; Sodium: 59mg; Protein: 4g

WATERCRESS, ORANGE AND CRANBERRY SALAD

SERVES 2 / PREP TIME: 5 MINUTES / COOK TIME: N/A

Fruity fun and fast!

---

2 TBSP BALSAMIC VINEGAR

4 TSP EXTRA VIRGIN OLIVE OIL

1/2 CUP FRESH CRANBERRIES

2 TSP FRESH GINGER, PEELED AND GRATED

A PINCH OF BLACK PEPPER TO TASTE

1 CUP FRESH WATERCRESS

1 ORANGE, PEELED AND SLICED

---

1. Grab a salad bowl and mix the vinegar and olive oil until blended and then add in the cranberries, ginger and pepper to taste
2. Add the watercress and orange slices to the dressing, and then toss to coat.
3. Chill for 15 minutes before serving.

Tip: Use grapefruit instead of orange if you have been advised not to include oranges in your diet - check with your doctor if unsure.

Per serving: Calories: 304; Fat: 27g; Carbohydrates: 15g; Phosphorus: 57g; Potassium: 392mg; Sodium: 33mg; Protein: 2g

ZUCCHINI AND CRISPY SALMON SALAD

SERVES 2 / PREP TIME: 2 MINUTES / COOK TIME: 15 MINUTES

Superb salad dish.

---

4 OZ SKINLESS SALMON FILLETS

2 TBSP EXTRA VIRGIN OLIVE OIL

1 LEMON, JUICED

1/2 CUP ZUCCHINI, SLICED

1/2 CUP OF SPINACH

1 TBSP BALSAMIC VINEGAR

2 SPRIGS THYME, TORN FROM THE STEM

---

1. Preheat the broiler on a medium to high heat.
2. Cook the salmon in parchment paper with 1 tbsp. oil and lemon for 10 minutes.
3. Remove the parchment paper and finish under the broiler for 5 minutes until golden brown and crispy.
4. Remove.
5. Heat 1 tbsp. oil in a pan on a medium heat.
6. Add the zucchini slices and sauté for 5-6 minutes.
7. Add the spinach to the pan and allow to wilt for 30 seconds.
8. Add salmon fillets to a bed of zucchini and spinach and drizzle with balsamic vinegar and a sprinkle of thyme.

Per serving: Calories: 226; Fat: 16g; Carbohydrates: 5g; Phosphorus: 189mg; Potassium: 396mg; Sodium: 238mg; Protein: 15g

RAINBOW RICE SALAD

SERVES 4 / PREP TIME: 10 MINUTES / COOK TIME: 35 MINUTES
Tasty colorful rice side dish.

1 TBSP EXTRA VIRGIN OLIVE OIL

2 TBSP BALSAMIC VINEGAR

1 TSP BLACK PEPPER

1 GARLIC CLOVE, MINCED

1 TSP DRIED BASIL

1 TSP DRIED OREGANO

1 TSP FRESH PARSLEY

1 RED BELL PEPPER, DICED

1/2 RED ONION, DICED

1/4 CUCUMBER, PEELED AND DICED

1 1/2 CUPS COOKED BROWN/WHITE RICE

1/2 CUP COOKED GREEN BEANS, CHOPPED

1. Add all the ingredients to a bowl and toss to coat (ensure cooked rice is completely cool).
2. Add to an airtight container and store in the fridge for up to 2 days.
3. Serve cold.

Tip: Check with your dietitian as to whether they recommend brown or white rice for your personalised dietary needs.

Per serving: Calories: 145; Fat: 3g; Carbohydrates: 25g; Phosphorus: 85mg; Potassium: 179g; Sodium: 8mg; Protein: 3g

TURNIP AND RUTABAGA MASH

SERVES 2 / PREP TIME: 10 MINUTES / COOK TIME: 20 MINUTES

Try this home comfort with a little twist!

3/4 CUP RUTABAGA, PEELED AND CHOPPED

2 TURNIPS, PEELED AND CHOPPED

2 TBSP TARRAGON, FINELY CHOPPED

1 TBSP EXTRA VIRGIN OLIVE OIL

A PINCH OF BLACK PEPPER

---

1. Soak vegetables in warm water for 10 minutes.
2. Add the rutabaga and turnip to a large pan of water, bring to the boil, and cook for 15-20 minutes until vegetables very soft.
3. Drain and add the tarragon and olive oil to the vegetables and season with pepper.
4. Mash in a separate bowl using a potato masher or fork.
5. Serve hot!

Per serving: Calories: 103; Fat: 7g; Carbohydrates: 9g; Phosphorus: 56mg; Potassium: 364mg; Sodium: 23mg; Protein: 2g

CURRIED COUSCOUS

SERVES 2 / PREP TIME: 5 MINUTES / COOK TIME: 20 MINUTES

Spicy and delicious side dish.

---

2 TBSP EXTRA VIRGIN OLIVE OIL

1 GREEN ONION, DICED

2 CLOVES GARLIC, MINCED

1 CUP COUSCOUS

1 CUP HOME-MADE CHICKEN STOCK (p. 52)

2 CUPS WATER

1 TBSP CURRY POWDER

1 TBSP CHILI POWDER

---

1. Heat the oil in a large pan on a medium heat, adding in the onions and garlic and sautéing for 2 minutes or until soft.
2. Add in the couscous and stir until lightly toasted.
3. Add the stock and water to the pan and boil on a high heat before reducing heat and adding in the curry and chili powders.
4. Cover and simmer for 20 minutes or until the couscous has soaked up most of the liquid.
5. Use your fork to stir through the couscous and serve with your favorite meat, fish or vegetable entrée.

Per serving: Calories: 220; Fat: 15g; Carbohydrates: 20g; Phosphorus: 43mg; Potassium: 194mg; Sodium: 176mg; Protein: 4g

STRAWBERRY AND MINT FRUIT SALAD

SERVES 2 / PREP TIME: 5 MINUTES / COOK TIME: N/A

A refreshing sweet and savory salad.

---

1 CUP STRAWBERRIES, SLICED

1 TBSP FRESH MINT, FINELY CHOPPED

1 TSP BALSAMIC VINEGAR

---

1. Mix all ingredients in a bowl and serve right away.

Per serving: Calories: 26; Fat: 0g; Carbohydrates: 6g; Phosphorus: 18mg; Potassium: 118mg; Sodium: 2mg; Protein: 1g

BRIE AND APPLE SALAD

SERVES 2 / PREP TIME: 5 MINUTES / COOK TIME: N/A

Peppery and sweet at the same time.

---

1 CUP WATERCRESS

1 TSP WHITE WINE VINEGAR

1/2 CUP BRIE, SLICED

1/2 APPLE, PEELED, CORED AND DICED

---

1. Toss watercress in vinegar and scatter with brie and apple.
2. Serve with Melba toast or crackers.

Per serving: Calories: 80, Fat: 5g; Carbohydrates: 5g; Phosphorus: 48mg; Potassium: 120mg; Sodium: 121mg; Protein: 4g

STOCKS AND SAUCES

BEETROOT SAUCE

SERVES 4 / PREP TIME: 10 MINUTES / COOK TIME: N/A

A delicious homemade condiment to dip your vegetable chips or crudités into!

---

1 CUP OF CANNED BEETROOT, NO ADDED SUGAR OR SALT

1 JUICED LEMON

1 TSP DRY MUSTARD

A PINCH OF BLACK PEPPER TO TASTE

---

1. Add all of the ingredients to a blender and purée until smooth.
2. Serve immediately or store in an airtight container in the fridge for 2-3 days.
3. Tastes great with homemade turnip chips or eggplant fries.

Per serving: Calories: 22; Fat: 0g; Carbohydrates: 5g; Phosphorus: 18mg; Potassium: 143mg; Sodium: 47mg; Protein: 1g

HOT SAUCE

SERVES 5 / PREP TIME: 5 MINUTES / COOK TIME: 20 MINUTES

A great sauce to add to any BBQ, snack or meal!

2 TBSP CANOLA OIL

1 TBSP ALL-PURPOSE WHITE FLOUR

1/4 CUP TARRAGON VINEGAR

1/4 CUP ONION, FINELY DICED

1 CUP WATER

2 TSP DRY MUSTARD

1 TSP CHILI POWDER

1. Mix oil and flour together to make a paste before adding the rest of the ingredients and transferring to a pan.
2. Cook the mixture for 15-20 minutes over a low heat until it starts to thicken.
3. Sauce can be used to brush on meats, fish or vegetables before cooking.

Per serving: Calories: 64; Fat: 6g; Carbohydrates: 3g; Phosphorus: 10mg; Potassium: 36mg; Sodium: 47mg; Protein: 0g

HOMEMADE PORK GRAVY

SERVES 5 / PREP TIME: 5 MINUTES / COOK TIME: 25 MINUTES

A healthy gravy to go with your roast. Remember to count your sauces and gravies towards your daily nutrition tracking!

1 TSP GROUND SAGE	6 OZ LEAN GROUND PORK, MINCED
1 TSP GROUND BASIL	2 CUPS WATER
1 TSP BLACK PEPPER	1 TBSP CORNSTARCH
a	
1 TSP FENNEL SEEDS	
1 TSP PAPRIKA	

1. Combine the herbs and spices with the ground pork.
2. Add a pot to the stove on a medium to high heat and cook the pork mix for 15 minutes or until cooked through.
3. Add the water and cornstarch to the pot and turn the heat down to simmer for a further 10 minutes.
4. Blend in a food processor until liquid consistency is reached and strain to get rid of any lumps.
5. Seal in an airtight container once cool to use a gravy for meats.

Per serving: Calories: 114; Fat: 7g; Carbohydrates: 3g; Phosphorus: 85mg; Potassium: 196mg; Sodium: 145mg; Protein: 9g

WHITE CHEESE SAUCE

SERVES 5 / PREP TIME: 5 MINUTES / COOK TIME: 20 MINUTES

To be used with lasagna, pastas or over pork and fish. Remember to count towards your daily nutrition tracking!

---

1 TBSP UNSALTED BUTTER

1/4 CUP ALL PURPOSE WHITE FLOUR

3/4 CUP 1% LOW-FAT MILK/RICE MILK (UNENRICHED)

4 OZ CREAM CHEESE

1/2 CUP BRIE

1/4 TSP WHITE PEPPER

1 TSP BLACK PEPPER

---

1. Heat saucepan on a medium heat.
2. Add the butter to the pan on the side nearest to the handle.
3. Tilt the pan towards you and allow butter to melt, whilst trying not to let it cover the rest of the pan.
4. Now add the flour to the opposite side of the pan and gradually mix the flour into the butter - continue to mix until smooth.
5. Add the milk and stir thoroughly for 10 minutes until lumps dissolve.
6. Add the cheese (optional) and stir for a further 5 minutes.
7. Turn off the heat, sprinkle with pepper and serve immediately.

Per serving: Calories: 186; Fat: 14g; Carbohydrates: 8g; Phosphorus: 94mg; Potassium: 122mg; Sodium: 190mg; Protein: 6g

SPICY MANGO CHUTNEY

SERVES 4 / PREP TIME: 5 MINUTES / COOK TIME: 15 MINUTES

Great as a dip, with curries or even as a salad topper.

---

1 TBSP CANOLA OIL

1/2 CUP ONION, FINELY DICED

2 TSP FRESH GINGER ROOT, MINCED

1 CUP MANGO, FINELY DICED

1 TSP CHILI POWDER

1 TSP CUMIN

---

1. Heat the oil in a skillet over a medium to high heat.
2. Sauté onion for 5 minutes until soft.
3. Add the ginger and stir for 2 minutes.
4. Now add the rest of the ingredients, cover and turn down the heat.
5. Simmer for 10-15 minutes.
6. Remove from heat to cool.
7. Store in an airtight container in the fridge for 2-3 days.

Per serving: Calories: 63; Fat: 4g; Carbohydrates: 8g; Phosphorus: 18mg; Potassium: 113mg; Sodium: 29mg; Protein: 1g

HONEY AND MUSTARD DRESSING

SERVES 2 / PREP TIME: 5 MINUTES / COOK TIME: N/A

A lovely fresh dressing for salads, vegetables or over meats and fish.

1 TBSP FRENCH MUSTARD

1 TBSP HONEY

1 TBSP EXTRA VIRGIN OLIVE OIL

1. Whisk all ingredients in a bowl until combined.
2. Cover and store in the refrigerator for up to 1 week.

Per serving: Calories: 95; Fat: 7g; Carbohydrates: 9g; Phosphorus: 6mg; Potassium: 12mg; Sodium: 57mg; Protein: 0g

CAJUN SPICE RUB

SERVES 2 / PREP TIME: 5 MINUTES / COOK TIME: N/A

Great as a dip, with curries or even as a salad topper.

---

1 GARLIC CLOVE, MINCED

2 TSP BLACK PEPPER

2 TSP CAYENNE PEPPER

1 TSP CHILI POWDER

2 TSP DRIED THYME

2 TSP DRIED OREGANO

---

1. Mix all ingredients together and store in an airtight container in a dry place.
2. Use as a rub for meats and fishes before cooking.

Per serving: Calories: 25; Fat: 1g; Carbohydrates: 5g; Phosphorus: 20mg; Potassium: 159mg ; Sodium: 112mg; Protein: 1g

SWEET CHILI AND LIME

SERVES 4 / PREP TIME: 5 MINUTES / COOK TIME: 7 MINUTES

A lovely sweet and savory sauce that can be used as a marinade or condiment

1 LIME

1/4 CUP CORNSTARCH

1/2 CUP WATER

2 GARLIC CLOVES

1 RED JALAPEÑO CHILI PEPPER

2 TBSP WHITE WINE VINEGAR

2 TBSP BROWN SUGAR

1. Reserve the lime, cornstarch and water.
2. Mix the rest of the ingredients in a blender or food processor until smooth.
3. Add the mixture to a pan on a medium to high heat and leave for 5 minutes until it starts to thicken.
4. Now add the cornstarch, juice of 1 lime and 2 tablespoons water to loosen the mixture a little for a further 2 minutes.
5. Remove from heat to cool.
6. Store in an airtight container in the fridge for 2-3 days.

Per serving: Calories: 15; Fat: 0g; Carbohydrates: 4g; Phosphorus: 6mg; Potassium: 35mg; Sodium: 3mg; Protein: 0g

MIXED HERB MARINADE

SERVES 5 / PREP TIME: 5 MINUTES / COOK TIME: NA

A handy dry mix that can be quickly added to oil to use as a marinade.

---

1 TSP BLACK PEPPER

1 GARLIC CLOVE, MINCED

1 CELERY STALK, MINCED

2 TSP MUSTARD SEEDS, CRUSHED

1 TSP DRIED BASIL

1 TSP DRIED THYME

1 TSP DRIED OREGANO

---

1. Combine all ingredients in a food processor until a fine powder is formed.
2. Store in an airtight container in a dry place.
3. When ready to use, mix with 1 tbsp. olive oil and baste meats/fish/vegetables or alternatively use as a dry rub for broiling.

Per serving: Calories: 9; Fat: 0g; Carbohydrates: 1g; Phosphorus: 11mg; Potassium: 46mg; Sodium: 7mg; Protein: 0g

WILD GARLIC PESTO

SERVES 5 / PREP TIME: 5 MINUTES / COOK TIME: NA

Delicious kidney friendly pesto!

1/2 CUP FRESH BASIL

1/2 CUP FRESH SPINACH/ARUGULA

1 TSP BLACK PEPPER

1/4 CUP EXTRA VIRGIN OLIVE OIL

1/4 CUP OF WILD GARLIC LEAVES (2 GARLIC CLOVES AS ALTERNATIVE)

1 LEMON, JUICED

1. Blend all ingredients in a food processor or a blender to reach required texture - chunky for a rustic feel or smooth as a dressing.
2. Store in an airtight container in the fridge for 3-4 days.
3. Serve over pasta, roasted vegetables, or as a dip for your favorite raw veg!

Per serving: Calories: 102; Fat: 11g; Carbohydrates: 1g; Phosphorus: 7mg; Potassium: 48mg; Sodium: 3mg; Protein: 0g

MEXICAN SALSA

SERVES 2 / PREP TIME: 5 MINUTES / COOK TIME: NA

Refreshing and vibrant.

1/4 RED ONION, FINELY DICED

1 LIME, JUICED

1/2 LEMON, JUICED

1 TSP WHITE VINEGAR

1 TSP BLACK PEPPER

1/4 CUP MANGO/PINEAPPLE, DICED

1 TBSP FRESH CILANTRO, FINELY CHOPPED

---

1. Soak vegetables in warm water prior to use.
2. Combine all ingredients in a bowl and toss to coat.
3. Store in an airtight container in the fridge for 2-3 days or serve right away.
4. Use on the side of fish, meats, tacos or salads.

Per serving: Calories: 35; Fat: 0g; Carbohydrates: 9g; Phosphorus: 18mg; Potassium: 134mg; Sodium: 2mg; Protein: 1g

DRINKS AND DESSERTS

SCRUMPTIOUS STRAWBERRY SMOOTHIE

SERVES 2 / PREP TIME: 5 MINUTES / COOK TIME: N/A

A healthy strawberry milkshake that everyone can enjoy!

1 CUP FRESH STRAWBERRIES, SLICED

1 CUP RICE MILK, UNENRICHED

1. Blend in a food processor or smoothie maker and serve over ice if desired.
2. Enjoy!

Per serving: Calories: 80; Fat: 2g; Carbohydrates: 12g; Phosphorus: 73mg; Potassium: 276mg; Sodium: 58mg; Protein: 4g

GINGER & LEMON GREEN ICED-TEA

SERVES 2 / PREP TIME: 5 MINUTES / COOK TIME: N/A

Refreshing iced-tea drink.

---

2 CUPS CONCENTRATED GREEN OR
MACHA TEA, SERVED HOT

1 LEMON, CUT INTO WEDGES

1/4 CUP CRYSTALLIZED GINGER,
CHOPPED INTO FINE PIECES

---

1. Get a glass container and mix the tea with the ginger and then cover and chill for 3 hours.
2. Strain and pour into serving glasses on top of ice if you wish.
3. Garnish with a wedge of lemon to serve.

Per serving: Calories: 20; Fat: 0g; Carbohydrates: 5g; Phosphorus: 9mg; Potassium: 106mg; Sodium: 4mg; Protein: 1g

LEMON SMOOTHIE

SERVES 2 / PREP TIME: 5 MINUTES / COOK TIME: N/A

Such a refreshing drink!

---

2 TBSP LEMON JUICE

2 TBSP BROWN SUGAR OR STEVIA

4 PASTEURIZED LIQUID EGG WHITES

---

1. Combine all ingredients in a blender until smooth.
2. Garnish with a slice of lemon.

Per serving: Calories: 49; Fat: 0g; Carbohydrates: 5g; Phosphorus: 10mg; Potassium: 112mg ; Sodium: 110mg; Protein: 8g

TROPICAL JUICE

SERVES 2 / PREP TIME: 5 MINUTES / COOK TIME: N/A

Tastes delicious on a hot Summer's day.

2 CUPS FRESH PINEAPPLE, PEELED AND
CUT INTO CHUNKS.

1/2 CUP LOW FAT COCONUT MILK

1 CUP WATER

1. Add all ingredients to your juicer and blend until smooth.
2. Serve immediately.

Tip: Check with your doctor or dietitian as to whether you can still have coconut milk. Alternatively use a non-dairy milk such as almond.

Per serving: Calories: 55; Fat: 9g; Carbohydrates: 6g; Phosphorus: 11mg; Potassium: 129mg; Sodium: 111mg; Protein: 7g

MIXED FRUIT ANTI-INFLAMMATORY SMOOTHIE

SERVES 4 / PREP TIME: 5 MINUTES / COOK TIME: N/A

This delectable smoothie is full of powerful antioxidants.

1 CUP RED OR WHITE GRAPES

1 CUP SLICED FROZEN OR FRESH PEACHES

1 CUP CHOPPED CABBAGE

1/2 CUP ICE CUBES

1/2 CUP WATER

1 SPRIG OF FRESH MINT

1. Toss all of the ingredients in a blender or juicer and blend until smooth.
2. Serve immediately in tall glasses.
3. Tear mint with fingers and serve with smoothies (optional).

Per serving: Calories: 48; Fat: 0g; Carbohydrates: 12g; Phosphorus: 17mg; Potassium: 203mg ; Sodium: 6mg; Protein: 1g

BANANA APPLE SMOOTHIE

SERVES 4 / PREP TIME: 5 MINUTES / COOK TIME: N/A

A breakfast or mid meal treat – this will taste excellent and keep you going until your next meal.

---

1 BANANA

1 APPLE, CORED AND PEELED

2 CUPS FILTERED WATER

1 TBSP STEVIA

1 CUP LOW FAT COCONUT MILK

---

1. Take a food processor and add all of the ingredients, processing until smooth.
2. Serve over ice.

Tip: Check with your doctor or dietitian as to whether you can still have coconut milk. Alternatively use a non-dairy milk such as almond.

Per serving: Calories: 182; Fat: 14g; Carbohydrates: 16g; Phosphorus: 70mg; Potassium: 300mg; Sodium: 14mg; Protein: 2g

WINTER BERRY ICED MILKSHAKE

SERVES 4 / PREP TIME: 5 MINUTES / COOK TIME: N/A

Rich in color and nutrients.

---

1 CUP RICE MILK, UNENRICHED

1/2 CUP ORGANIC BLUEBERRIES (OR WASHED IF NON-ORGANIC)

1/2 CUP BLACKBERRIES

ICE CUBES TO DESIRED CONCENTRATION

---

1. Add ingredients together in a blender, blending until smooth and then serve in tall glasses.

Per serving: Calories: 45; Fat: 1g; Carbohydrates: 7g; Phosphorus: 33mg; Potassium: 118mg; Sodium: 29mg; Protein: 2g

COCONUT PANCAKES

SERVES 2 / PREP TIME: 5 MINUTES / COOK TIME: 10 MINUTES

Tropical dessert.

---

2 FREE RANGE EGG WHITES

2 TBSP ALL PURPOSE WHITE FLOUR

3 TBSP COCONUT SHAVINGS

2 TBSP COCONUT MILK (OPTIONAL)

1 TBSP COCONUT OIL

---

1. Get a bowl and combine all the ingredients.
2. Mix well until you get a thick batter.
3. Heat a skillet on a medium heat and heat the coconut oil.
4. Pour half the mixture to the center of the pan, forming a pancake and cook through for 3-4 minutes on each side.
5. Serve with your choice of berries on the top.

Tip: Check with your doctor or dietitian as to whether you can still have coconut milk. Alternatively use a non-dairy milk such as almond.

Per serving: Calories: 177; Fat: 13g; Carbohydrates: 12g; Phosphorus: 37mg; Potassium: 133mg; Sodium: 133mg; Protein: 5g

SPICED PEACHES

SERVES 2 / PREP TIME: 5 MINUTES / COOK TIME: 10 MINUTES

These are so easy to prepare and impress every time.

---

1 CUP CANNED PEACHES IN THEIR OWN JUICES

1/2 TSP CORNSTARCH

1 TSP GROUND CLOVES

1 TSP GROUND CINNAMON

1 TSP GROUND NUTMEG

ZEST OF 1/2 LEMON

1/2 CUP WATER

---

1. Drain peaches.
2. Combine water, cornstarch, cinnamon, nutmeg, ground cloves and lemon zest in a pan on the stove.
3. Heat on a medium heat and add peaches.
4. Bring to a boil, reduce the heat and simmer for 10 minutes.
5. Serve warm.

Per serving: Calories: 70; Fat: 1g; Carbohydrates: 18g; Phosphorus: 26mg; Potassium: 184mg; Sodium: 9mg; Protein: 1g

PUMPKIN CHEESECAKE BAR

SERVES 4 / PREP TIME: 10 MINUTES / COOK TIME: 50 MINUTES

A scrumptious piece of indulgence - Enjoy low sodium canned pumpkin in early stages of kidney disease and always check with your doctor.

2 1/2 TBSP UNSALTED BUTTER

4 OZ CREAM CHEESE

1/2 CUP ALL-PURPOSE WHITE FLOUR

3 TBSP GOLDEN BROWN SUGAR

1/4 CUP GRANULATED SUGAR

1/2 CUP PURÉED PUMPKIN

2 EGG WHITES

1 TSP GROUND CINNAMON

1 TSP GROUND NUTMEG

1 TSP VANILLA EXTRACT

1. Preheat the oven to 350°f/170°c/Gas Mark 4.
2. Remove butter and cream cheese from the fridge.
3. Mix the flour and brown sugar in a mixing bowl.
4. Mix in the butter with your fingertips to form 'breadcrumbs'.
5. Place 3/4 of this mixture into the bottom of an ovenproof dish.
6. Bake in the oven for 15 minutes and remove to cool.
7. Lightly whisk the egg and fold in the cream cheese, sugar (or substitute stevia), pumpkin, cinnamon, nutmeg, and vanilla until smooth.
8. Pour this mixture over the oven-baked base and sprinkle with the rest of the breadcrumbs from earlier.
9. Place back in the oven and bake for a further 30-35 minutes.
10. Allow to cool and slice to serve.

Per serving: Calories: 296; Fat: 17g; Carbohydrates: 30g; Phosphorus: 62mg; Potassium: 164g; Sodium: 159mg; Protein: 5g

BLUEBERRY AND VANILLA MINI MUFFINS

SERVES 5 / PREP TIME: 10 MINUTES / COOK TIME: 35 MINUTES

Scrumptious muffins to be enjoyed as a delicious dessert or breakfast!

---

3 EGG WHITES

1/4 CUP ALL PURPOSE WHITE FLOUR

1 TBSP COCONUT FLOUR

1 TSP OF BAKING SODA

1 TBSP NUTMEG, GRATED

1 TSP VANILLA EXTRACT

1 TSP STEVIA

1/4 CUP FRESH BLUEBERRIES

---

1. Pre-heat the oven to 325°F/170 °C/Gas Mark 3.
2. Mix all of the ingredients in a mixing bowl.
3. Divide the batter into 4 and spoon into a lightly oiled muffin tin.
4. Bake in the oven for 15-20 minutes or until cooked through.
5. Your knife should pull out clean from the middle of the muffin once done.
6. Allow to cool on a wired rack before serving.

Per serving: Calories: 48; Fat: 1g; Carbohydrates: 8g; Phosphorus: 14mg; Potassium: 44mg; Sodium: 298mg; Protein: 2g

CONVERSION TABLES

Volume

Imperial	Metric
1 tbsp	15ml
2 fl oz	55 ml
3 fl oz	75 ml
5 fl oz (¼ pint)	150 ml
10 fl oz (½ pint)	275 ml
1 pint	570 ml
1 ¼ pints	725 ml
1 ¾ pints	1 liter
2 pints	1.2 liters
2½ pints	1.5 liters
4 pints	2.25 liters

Oven temperatures

Gas Mark	Fahrenheit	Celsius
1/4	225	110
1/2	250	130
1	275	140
2	300	150
3	325	170
4	350	180
5	375	190
6	400	200
7	425	220
8	450	230
9	475	240

Weight

Imperial	Metric
½ oz	10 g
¾ oz	20 g
1 oz	25 g
1½ oz	40 g
2 oz	50 g
2½ oz	60 g
3 oz	75 g
4 oz	110 g
4½ oz	125 g
5 oz	150 g
6 oz	175 g
7 oz	200 g
8 oz	225 g
9 oz	250 g
10 oz	275 g

BIBLIOGRAPHY

Garrick, R. (2008) 'Prevalence of chronic kidney disease in the United States', Yearbook of Medicine, 2008, pp. 215–217. doi: 10.1016/s0084-3873(08)79151-x.

Coresh, J., Astor, B.C., Greene, T., Eknoyan, G. and Levey, A.S. (2003) 'Prevalence of chronic kidney disease and decreased kidney function in the adult US population: Third national health and nutrition examination survey', American Journal of Kidney Diseases, 41(1), pp. 1–12. doi: 10.1053/ajkd.2003.50007.

Kopple, J.D. (2001) 'National kidney foundation K/DOQI clinical practice guidelines for nutrition in chronic renal failure', American Journal of Kidney Diseases, 37(1), pp. S66–S70. doi: 10.1053/ajkd.2001.20748.

Wilhelm-Leen, E.R., Hall, Y.N., Tamura, M.K. and Chertow, G.M. (2009) 'Frailty and chronic kidney disease: The Third national health and nutrition evaluation survey', The American Journal of Medicine, 122(7), pp. 664–671.e2. doi: 10.1016/j.amjmed.2009.01.026

Kidney Disease Outcomes Quality Initiative (K/DOQI) and the Dialysis Outcomes and Practice Patterns Study (DOPPS): Nutrition guidelines, indicators, and practices

Kalantar-Zadeh, K., Gutekunst, L., Mehrotra, R., Kovesdy, C.P., Bross, R., Shinaberger, C.S., Noori, N., Hirschberg, R., Benner, D., Nissenson, A.R. and Kopple, J.D. (2010) 'Understanding sources of dietary phosphorus in the treatment of patients with chronic kidney disease', Clinical Journal of the American Society of Nephrology, 5(3), pp. 519–530. doi: 10.2215/cjn.06080809.

Epstein, F.H., Brenner, B.M., Meyer, T.W. and Hostetter, T.H. (1982) 'Dietary protein intake and the progressive nature of kidney disease:', New England Journal of Medicine, 307(11), pp. 652–659. doi: 10.1056/nejm198209093071104.

Research, K. (2016) Kidney research UK - kidney research UK. Available at: https://www.kidneyresearchuk.org/health-information/chronic-kidney-disease (Accessed: 25 March 2016).

Foundation, N.K. (2014) Nutrition. Available at: https://www.kidney.org/nutrition (Accessed: 20 February 2016).

nc, D.H.P. (2004) Top 15 healthy foods for people with kidney disease. Available at: https://www.davita.com/kidney-disease/diet-and-nutrition/lifestyle/top-15-healthy-foods-for-people-with-kidney-disease/e/5347 (Accessed: 25 July 2016).

INDEX

Made in the USA
San Bernardino, CA
23 April 2018